Praise for *The Scoliosis Self-Help Resource Book*

"My congratulations to Dr. Esagui on the development of a direct and easy to use reference for persons seeking to learn more about the concept of scoliosis, chiropractic and self-care. In addition to the basics Dr. Esagui has provided information to assist with many other lifestyles issues that may impact on the circumstances related to scoliosis that are both informative and useful."

Dr. Gerard Clum, DC President of Life Chiropractic College West. CA

"Dr. Esagui has written an excellent guide for patients with scoliosis. Her book provides daily exercises (The Esagui Scoliosis Protocol – TESP) diet and lifestyle changes in order to combat scoliosis and its possible deleterious effects. This comprehensive resource allows patients to be proactive in managing their condition and gain a greater understanding of the pathophysiology of scoliosis. I highly recommend *The Scoliosis Self-Help Resource Book.*"

Dr. Jordi X. Kellogg, Specializing in the Treatment of Brain and Spinal Disorders.
Neurological Surgery, Portland, OR

"Dr. Esagui, I am so happy I found your book. I have several teenage patients with scoliosis and I was unable to find any reliable resource information to study or give to them. Your book was exactly what I was looking for. Thank you."

Dr. Diane Bellwood, DC Rancho Cucamonga, CA

"In this book Dr. Esagui presents simple solutions to very complex problems. She is a very gifted creative thinker who has translated her ideas into a concise and practical guide to scoliosis management. A must read for patients and doctors alike."

Dr. Neil McMahon, RN., DC, Oregon City, OR

"As a nutrition expert, I love that Dr. Veronica Esagui addresses what in my opinion is the true cornerstone to having lifelong optimal health. *The Scoliosis Self-Help Resource Book* educates the reader that it is possible to heal yourself through healthy eating, proper exercises and taking into account the big picture of health, including such things as sleep and stress. Quotes in the book such as "Most of our present health is in alignment to our way of life" provides great motivation to the reader."

Lila Ojeda, MS,RD,LD,CSCS Registered Dietitian & Personal Trainer.
Specializing in Yoga and Pilates. Lake Oswego, OR www.LO-Solutions.com

"*The Scoliosis Self-Help Resource Book* by Dr. Veronica Esagui, is a true inspirational resource for anyone wanting to find out how to improve the curvature of their spine and improve their overall health."

Ashley Pennewill, Publisher, Natural Awakenings Magazine. Portland, OR

"Tigard chiropractor writes holistic scoliosis book" an interview with Dr. Veronica Esagui was featured in The Times, Tigard, OR November 21, 2008.
"The Scoliosis Self-Help Resource Book" was featured in The American Chiropractor Magazine December 2008 Volume 30, number 12.

The
Scoliosis
Self-Help Resource Book

Includes The Illustrated Step-By-Step Approach to The Esagui Scoliosis Protocol (TESP)

Dr. Veronica Esagui, Chiropractic Physician

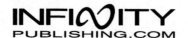

Copyright © 2008 by Dr. Veronica Esagui

The descriptions of medical conditions are based solely on publicly available information. In certain instances, we have listed products by their brand names, as that is how they are known, and in order to provide relevant information for the reader. We have no connections to any of the companies or brand-name products listed in this book.

The information in this book should not be used as a substitute for advice from a qualified health-care practitioner. In the event you use the information in this book without a health care practitioner's approval, you are prescribing for yourself, which is your constitutional right, but the author assumes no responsibility. See your chiropractor for diagnosis and treatment of any medical concerns you may have, or before implementing any diet, supplement, exercise or other lifestyle changes.

This book may be purchased for educational or sales promotional use.
21860 Willamette Drive
West Linn, OR 97068
(503) 650-2394
www.veronicaesagui.com

Technical Editors: Dr. Ralph Ezagui,
Dr. Pam Pavalonis
Editor: Chory Ferguson
Cover Graphic Designer: Laurie Ryan-Day,
Ryan Graphics

Photography: Dwon Güvenir
Text Design and Illustrations: Dr.Veronica Esagui
Front Cover Photograph (Model's Back) Danlar
Model's back, Front Cover: Cheryl Fitzpatrick
Poetry: Danlar

ISBN 0-7414-4647-2
Published by:

INFINITY
PUBLISHING.COM
1094 New DeHaven Street, Suite 100
West Conshohocken, PA 19428-2713
Info@buybooksontheweb.com
www.buybooksontheweb.com
Toll-free (877) BUY BOOK
Local Phone (610) 941-9999
Fax (610) 941-9959

Printed in the United States of America
Printed on Recycled Paper
Published January 2009

This book is dedicated to all my patients; particularly Jean, a 13 year old girl, who showed me that with strong commitment nothing is impossible.

I want to thank my son Dr. Ralph Esagui, for his collaboration and guidance through the writing process and for always being my true friend. I feel very privileged and honored that he is both my son and colleague.

I would like to thank my husband Dan, who stood by my side when I was ready to give up, making the process of writing this book a loving joint effort.

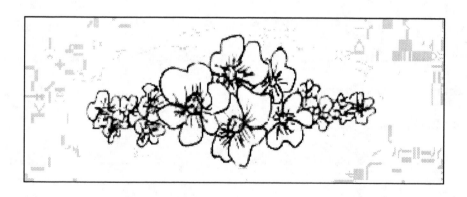

Table of Contents

The doctor of the future will give no medicine,
but will interest patients in the care of the human frame,
in diet, and in the cause and prevention of disease.

Thomas A. Edison

Preface

The first time I thought of writing about Scoliosis was in 2001, but that book would have been written out of frustration. I am glad I never wrote it. The reason for feeling that way was because of Sara, a 14-year-old girl who my son, Dr. Ralph, and I met while doing a health fair in Gladstone, Oregon.

We were using the Spinal Analysis Machine (SAM, measures the relative discrepancies in the spine, showing clearly, differences from one side of the body to the other) at the weekend fair, when we met Sara and her mom. They stopped by our tent and wanted us to evaluate Sara's back. After the spinal screening, we sat with both of them and explained that Sara needed chiropractic care, not only to help with the back pain, but also to help manage her condition and possibly slow down the progression of her Scoliosis. "Sara already has a real good doctor," her mother told us, "and he said she needs back surgery done by next month. Besides," she added with a joyful smile, "the insurance will cover the complete cost of the surgery. So why should we wait?"

We spent the next forty-five minutes trying to convince her to bring Sara to our office for further evaluation. We offered free chiropractic care for a year, if only she held-off on the surgery and gave her daughter and us a chance to try to make a difference in the outcome. My son went into full detail, explaining how serious and invasive the surgery was going to be. He poured his heart out in the hopes that Sara's mother would change her mind.

The next day, Sara came by our tent; "My mom spoke to my doctor and they are going to wait. I am not having surgery after all."

They never came to our office. I called their home once, in case they had lost our phone number, and left a message reminding them that our care was free of charge, and that we were looking forward to helping Sara.

A year later, we were back at the Gladstone Fair. Sara was at the fair grounds, and gave us the news. She was going to have back surgery in a few weeks.

It was heartbreaking for us that a whole year had gone by and no exercises had been given, no ergonomics, no diet, nothing had been attempted except for spine X-rays every three months, and the so-called "under observation" protocol of her orthopedic surgeon. When we asked her mom why she had opted to wait for surgery instead of trying something less invasive, she reminded us "Why not; the surgeon told us the insurance will cover the cost of surgery."

When my friend Lorraine, who lives in Portugal, told me that her son William was suffering from depression and anorexia, I was not surprised. He had been diagnosed with Scoliosis two years prior and since then had been under medical observation. He was told that he had to wear a body brace. William is 15 years old. Could this be the reason he had stopped eating? Could this be the reason for his depression? How is a 15 year-old boy supposed to feel when he is facing this kind of uncertainty? Besides being under medical observation, what had been done in those two years to help him cope with his future? Nothing except wait until the curvature of his spine would get bad enough to require back surgery.

Sara and William are only two of the many young people that have been told by the medical profession to wait and see what happens in the years ahead. I do not agree with that philosophy, it's about time everyone learns that there are other choices of care, which may slow down the progression of Scoliosis.

When Jean came to our office for the first time in July of 2006, she was 13 years old. Up to then, Jean had been under medical observation for Scoliosis. Several X-rays had been performed through the preceding years. She had never been shown her X-rays, but was aware there was something wrong with her back because of a constant dull backache.

The X-rays taken by Jean's doctor in December, 2005 showed that she had a lower back curve of 17 degrees and 8 degrees curve at the mid back. Four months later, in April of 2006, the next set of X-rays taken by her doctor showed the same 17 degrees at the lower back but the mid-back had increased to 12 degrees.

After taking her history and performing a spinal exam that included orthopedic and neurological testing, I referred Jean for a full spine X-Ray outside our office. She went to Dr Tyrone Wei, DACBR. The X-Rays were taken on August 2, 2006 and they were performed with Jean standing and without shoes. The new films showed the lower back curve had advanced to 20 degrees, mid-back to 16 degrees and lower part of the neck was now 14 degrees.

Jean's mom showed concern for her daughter's posture and, as she described it, "daily junk food addiction." I was concerned that, because of her age, Jean was not ready to make a lifestyle change. I needed her complete cooperation if the treatment plan was going to be successful. I reflected on my mother's teaching; "If you want someone to take an active part in solving a problem, you must show the evidence." So I did. Upon seeing her X-rays, Jean fainted.

It's not easy to make a teenager follow a specific protocol of exercises on a daily basis. As a matter of a fact, adults are no different. But Jean seemed eager to follow the treatment plan after having seen her X-rays. Besides chiropractic adjustments three times per week, ergonomics and diet were addressed. We talked about lifestyle changes and better habits. I felt so strongly about the regime of care being provided that I became inspired during this period to develop The Esagui Scoliosis Protocol (*TESP*) to help reverse Jean's spinal curvature, along with her chiropractic adjustments. Jean's parents kept her focused by providing plenty of love and persuasion. I had no doubt that this type of family involvement and commitment was going to be the essence of success.

Twice a day, Jean was to perform *TESP* at home. Sometimes, she would confess to skipping a day or two when *too* busy.

Still, her mom was amazed with the changes in Jean's lifestyle, "Jean still favors sweets, but she actually ate spinach today, and she is willing to eat healthier meals."

After eighteen weeks of chiropractic adjustments along with *TESP* Jean was referred out once again for a full spine X-ray at the end of December 2006.

***

Dr. Wei called to tell me the best news I could wish for Christmas: Jean's Scoliosis had improved considerably. The X-rays showed that the neck and upper back junction had decreased from 14 to 11 degrees, the thoracic region (mid-back) from 16 to 13 degrees, and the lumbar region (lower back) from 20 to 18 degrees.

Dr. Wei learned for the first time that I had been working on Jean's curvature for the last four months.

"Imagine!" he said with excitement, "If she achieved this type of improvement with chiropractic adjustments and following the exercises on an off and on basis, what would happen if she was to do them every single day, twice a day? Can you imagine what the results would have been, today?"

I agreed whole-heartedly with him.

The reality of life was a rude awakening for Jean and me on May 14, 2007 when her full spine X-ray was once again taken and the results proved that without motivation to continue exercising daily and to follow chiropractic treatment two to three times per week, the results can be devastating. Jean's X-rays were very clear, she had worsened; her neck and upper back junction had reversed to 14 degrees, the thoracic region had changed from 13 degrees to 15 degrees, and the lower back had gone from 18 degrees to 21 degrees.

I immediately blamed myself. I obviously had failed to instigate enough responsibility and enthusiasm in Jean to make her want to follow, the care she needed. Of course I also blamed Jean for assuming that her spine would just continue to correct itself, so she didn't have to work so hard at it. The afternoon I had spent in her home in the beginning of her treatment, going carefully over each specific exercise for her spine had been a waste of time. I felt the best thing I could do was to stop writing about the benefits of chiropractic and *TESP* since nobody seemed to care. I moped around the office that day feeling sorry for humankind and myself and for all the people that would continue to be told that there is no hope.

The medical model was right; nothing works because patients are not going to follow the care they need, it's easier to wait and have surgery when it gets bad enough. That's why some medical doctors send their patients to physical therapists who are nothing but personal trainers, making sure the patients exercise while being supervised like naughty little children. I can't go home with everybody, and nobody is going to come home with me so I can make sure they are exercising! The whole thing had been a lost cause and I waved my white flag to the enemy.

I was very grumpy when I went home that night and shared my *pity me* feelings, with my husband Dan who always listens to me when I have something bothering me. I told him what had happened and that I had decided not to waste any more time writing. I was dropping the project. I didn't expect his strong response.

"But, Veronica, can't you see that it did work? You have just proved it! Jean's curve did get better while she was following the treatment plan, and then she stopped so it got worse again. In other words, it doesn't work unless there is a firm dedication from the patient to continue with the treatment. You will be committing an injustice to everyone if you quit too." This statement made a lot of sense and jolted me back into action.

The next day I had to confront John, who is eighteen years old, and comes to our office once a week for his chiropractic adjustments. The first time he came to our office he was suffering from back pain due to severe forward curvature of the spine and mild Scoliosis. I had him on *TESP* and I had to find out if he was being compliant with home care. John is very proud of his new and improved posture and how good he looks since he started chiropractic a few months ago. I asked him if he was performing *TESP* daily.

He said, "Honestly, I did in the beginning for the first three months, but now that I can see that I am maintaining my spine straight, I stopped."

I told him what had happened to Jean when she stopped exercising daily and I had agreed she could come in just once a week for her adjustments. I was at fault for allowing her digression. I wanted to know how he felt; his opinion was important to me. I was afraid that if he stopped it was likely that his spine would get worse again, just like Jean.

"How can I get you motivated?" I asked him.

He said, "By not giving up on people like me. What you are doing is very important and it has made a difference in my life. Look at me; it worked."

If, by writing this book, I can shed some light on Scoliosis management that is more proactive than just waiting "under observation," then people will understand their options and I will have done my best as a chiropractor and educator.

I realize now that it is up to each individual to take responsibility for his or her life. But, one thing is for sure, without full commitment and perseverance, there are no satisfactory results.

Dr. Veronica Esagui

In life I cannot fail
when I learn.
Great decisions
blossom from experimentation.
Poor decisions build experience
as well as strength.

Danlar

Chiropractic Terms

Chiropractic – Is a primary health care profession that focuses on the anatomy of the spine, its immediate articulation, and the condition of nerve interference. It is based on the premise that good health depends in part upon a normally functioning nervous system.

Health – "A state of optimal physical, mental, and social well-being; and not merely the absence of disease and illness." – The World Health Organization.

Subluxation – Also referred to as nerve interference, is a word used by chiropractic physicians to describe a misalignment of one or more of the 24 vertebrae in the spinal column. See illustration on page 7 for a better understanding on how subluxations interfere with the nerves, the brain and the spinal cord's ability to function, affecting the health of our internal organs, muscles, and so on.

Adjustment – The specific application of forces used to correct subluxations (misalignment of the spine) and facilitate normal movement.

Vertebra – A single bone of the spinal column.

Vertebrae – More than one vertebra.

Disc – The cushion or pad in between the vertebrae. They act as shock absorbers to the spine, and give shape to the vertebral column.

Fixation – An area of the spine or specific joint with restricted motion.

Range of Motion – The amount of motion measured in degrees through which a joint may be moved.

Lateral – To the side.

Bilateral – To both sides.

Flexion – Bending forward.

Extension – Bending backwards.

Acute – Severe, rapid onset, short duration.

Chronic – Persisting for a long period of time.

Cervicals – The first seven vertebrae of the spinal column. The word *cervical* pertains to the neck.

Thoracics – The *thoracic vertebrae* lie in the posterior wall of the thorax. All twelve thoracic vertebrae have a pair of ribs attached to them.

Lumbars – The five *lumbar vertebrae* lie in the small of the back, below the thoracic vertebrae.

Sacrum – The triangular bone at the bottom of the spine.

Coccyx – The tailbone.

Infantile Scoliosis – Spinal curvature that develops during the first years of life. The earlier it develops, the more dangerous it is because there are more years for it to worsen.

Adolescent Scoliosis – Presence at or about the onset of puberty and before maturity (as early as 10 years old but before 25 years old).

Adult Scoliosis – Spinal curvature existing *after* skeletal maturity.

DextroScoliosis – The curve of the Scoliosis is directed to the *right* side of the body.

LevoScoliosis – The curve of the Scoliosis is directed to the *left* side of the body.

Correlative Spinal Anatomy: Douglas Gate D.C.
Terminology Committee, Scoliosis Society: A glossary of Scoliosis terms. Spine, 1:57, 1976.

The Function of the Spine

When a child comes to my office for care the first time, sometimes I will ask, "So, what do you think would happen to you, if you had no spine?" Some grasp the idea and say something like, "I would fall down?" and I add, "Like jelly on the floor."

The function of the spine, besides keeping us erect, is to house and protect the spinal cord, a very important part of our nervous system.

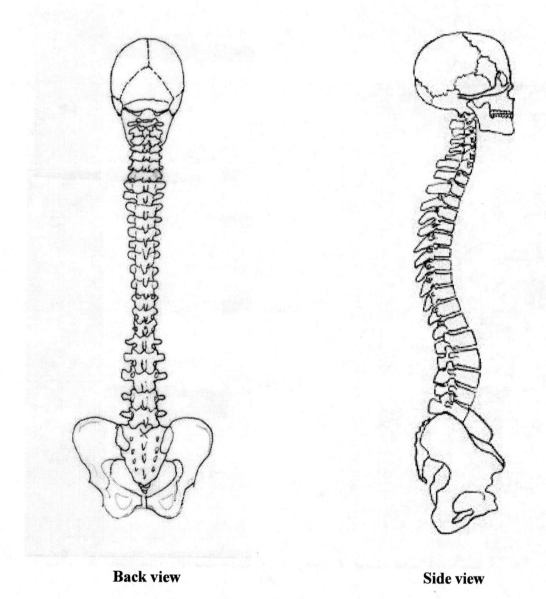

Back view   **Side view**

From the **back view**, the spine should look straight; from the neck, down to the triangular bone at the base of the spine called the sacrum.

Anatomy of the Spine

The spine consists of 24 movable vertebrae plus the sacrum and the coccyx.

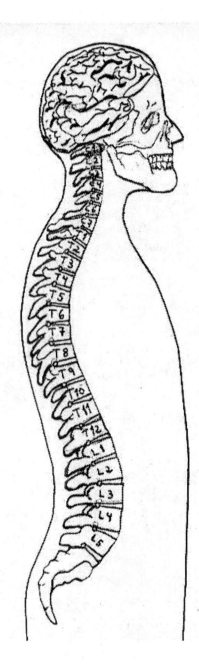

Brain
(Protected inside the skull)

Cervical spine
(Neck)
C1 through C7 (7 vertebrae)

Thoracic spine
(Back)
T1 through T12 (12 vertebrae)

Lumbar spine
(Lower back)
L1 through L5 (5 vertebrae)

Sacrum (5 fused vertebrae)

Coccyx Tailbone (4 fused vertebrae)

The bones that make up the spine
are called *vertebrae*

The *discs,* in between each vertebra,
can get worn out and bulge, pressing
painfully on nerves or the spinal cord itself.

When the vertebrae are not properly
aligned, it can press on the spinal
nerves which are between the vertebrae.

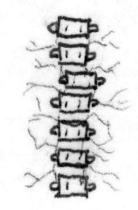

Should the above occur, the
muscles, (illustrated in gray)
will have to work harder to try
to balance the spine and can go
into spasms from being overused.
Sometimes, the spasm can be felt
on one side more than the other.

When the neck or the back are not
properly aligned (subluxation),
the natural curve is lost and will
naturally compensate by transferring
weight to the other side of the body.
    A good example would be the head,
which being on top of the spine, might
tend to bend more to one side than the
other, to compensate for the neck not
being aligned.
    The list goes on with every part of
our body. Check out page 5.

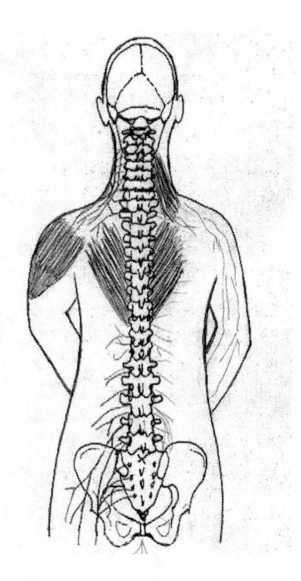

Scoliosis Facts

- Scoliosis is a sideways curve of the spine of 10 degrees or more and usually starts in childhood. It can make an "S" or "C" shape and sometimes causes stiffness and pain.

- If the curve is more than 60 degrees it is considered serious, because it can affect the lungs and if the curve is to the left side it can put pressure on the heart.

- Scoliosis comes from the Greek word skolios, which means "twisted or crooked."

- Scoliosis is not a disease, nor is it contagious.

- Mild forms occur equally in boys and girls but moderate to severe forms are more common in girls.

- *Idiopathic Scoliosis* is the term used to describe Scoliosis without a known cause.

- Some Scoliosis can only be seen upon bending forward, others make the waist or shoulders appear uneven.

- *Kyphosis* is another form of abnormal spinal curvature; instead of the spine bending sideways the spine bends forward.

- Drugs, pesticides, and herbicide exposure have been found to cause Scoliosis in animal studies.

- Scoliosis tends to occur between nine and fourteen years of age, when bones are growing the fastest.

- Early detection and management are very important to control the condition and prevent further complications.

- Outcomes depend on where and how much the spine curves, the patient's age, and when the symptoms appear. The greater the curve the more intense and challenging it becomes to address the condition.

- Idiopathic Scoliosis of more than 20 degrees presents a tenfold increase in the occurrences of congenital heart disease.[1]

[1] Reckles LN, Peterson HA, Bianco AJ, et al.: The association of Scoliosis and congenital heart disease. J Bone Joint Surg 57A: 449, 1975.

Two Types of Scoliosis

Nonstructural Scoliosis:

Postural: curvature resolves when lying down.

Compensatory: due to a leg-length difference; causes the hips and the spine to compensate by making the spine rotate or bend sideways but without rotation of the vertebra. A difference in leg length (one leg shorter than the other) can also produce Compensatory Scoliosis and misalignments, which are transferred upwards, distorting the lower back and the pelvis.

Chronic: constant, ongoing, or on-and-off; patient bends sideways to avoid impacting an irritated nerve like the sciatic nerve.

Structural Scoliosis: does not correct itself in the lying down position. It is more rigid.

Congenital: born with vertebrae that never developed properly. Abnormal vertebrae shapes can influence the spine curvature.

Neurogenic: spinal curvature caused by disease or anomaly of the nervous system. Some conditions, like cerebral palsy, infection, or tumors can cause Structural Scoliosis.

Idiopathic: No cause is established and it accounts for up to 80% of curvatures. Idiopathic Scoliosis is the least understood and can run in families; sometimes there is more than one member in the family with it.

Measure of Severity in Scoliosis

Mild to moderate..………17 degrees to 29 degrees of curvature

Moderate to severe…………………………………….30 degrees to 46 degrees or more of curvature

Scoliosis According to its Location

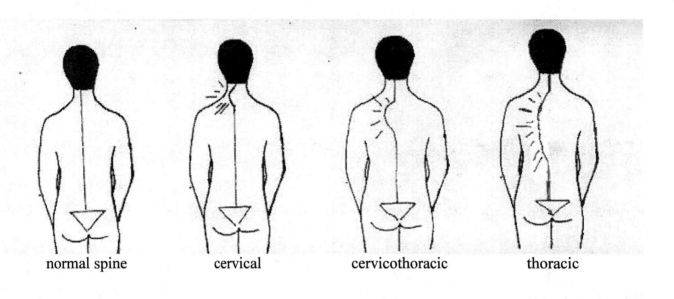

normal spine   cervical   cervicothoracic   thoracic

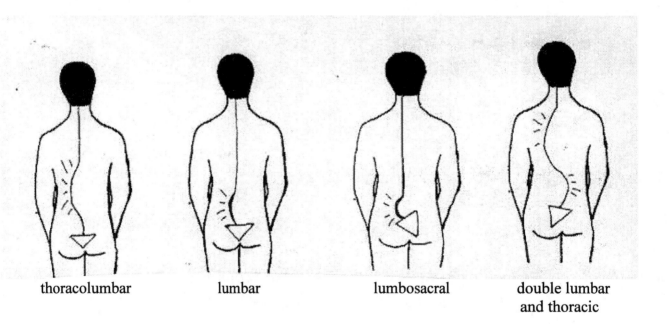

thoracolumbar   lumbar   lumbosacral   double lumbar and thoracic

The Nervous System and its Functions

If the nervous system controls the function of virtually every cell, tissue, and organ in our bodies, what happens when we have a subluxation interfering with the proper function of the nervous system?

This is a condensed version of where the nerves go, and what happens when a subluxation interferes with the nervous system and its proper function.

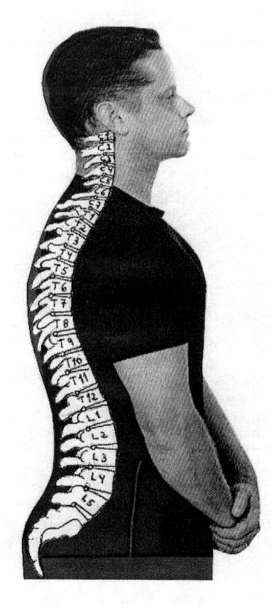

Nerve Function	Some **consequences from being subluxated**
C1 – Eyes, ears	Vision problems
C2 – Tongue, sinuses	Sinus problems
C3 – Teeth, outer ear	Hearing
C4 – Nose, lips, mouth	Headaches
C5 – Vocal chords, neck	Stiff neck
C7 – Thyroid gland, elbows	Upper arm pain
	Dizziness
	Hand/finger numbness
	Hand/finger pain
T1 – Heart, hands, arms	Tennis elbow
T2 – Coronary arteries	Shortness of breath
T3 – Chest, heart, lungs	Chest pain
T4 – Gallbladder	Gallbladder conditions
T5 – Liver	Liver conditions
T6 – Stomach	Indigestion
T7 – Pancreas, spleen	Heartburn
T8 – Adrenal cortex	Asthma
T9 – Ovaries, uterus	Sterility
T10 – Kidneys, testes	Blood pressure problems
T11 – Urinary bladder	Bed wetting
T12 – Lymph circulation	Fatigue
	Back pain
	Kidney conditions
	Gas pains
	Irritable bowel
L1 – Large intestine	Bladder problems
L2 – Abdomen, upper leg	Menstrual problems
L3 – Knees, sex organs	Knee pain
L4 – Sciatica nerve	Sciatica
L5 – Lower legs, feet	Poor circulation
	Radiating pain to legs
	Tingling feeling to feet
	Leg cramps/cold feet
	Numb feeling to legs/feet
Sacrum - Hip bones, genitalia	Sacroiliac problems
Coccyx - Rectum, anus	Lower back pain
	Hemorrhoids

The History of Chiropractic

As early as 2700 BC Hippocrates, the "father of medicine," used spinal manipulation to help patients with ailments.

Galen the Greek, a physician in Rome during the second century AD, and Ambroise Pare, the "father of surgery" in the 16th century, used techniques that had a striking resemblance to those used by chiropractors today. Many cultures referred to this form of treatment as "bone setting." This art was passed on through the centuries from one family member to another.

It wasn't until late 1800s, that Daniel D. Palmer – a self-taught healer in Davenport, Iowa – coined the term "chiropractic" which comes from the Greek words "hands on." This event happened one day when Harvey Lillard, a janitor working in Palmer's building, mentioned to Palmer that he had lost his hearing many years before when he was bending over and felt a "pop" in his upper back.

Daniel D. Palmer spent much of his time studying the structure of the spine and the ancient art of joint manipulation. He felt that the two events - the "popping" in Lillard's back and his deafness – were related. After examining Lillard's spine, Daniel D. Palmer found that one of the vertebrae was misaligned. He adjusted Lillard's vertebra into the correct position and an amazing event occurred. Lillard's hearing was restored! This famous *procedure* became known as a *chiropractic* adjustment; it was the solution to Daniel D. Palmer's goal at finding a cure for disease and illness that did not use drugs.

In 1898, Daniel D. Palmer opened the Palmer School & Infirmary of Chiropractic and began teaching his chiropractic techniques to others. Daniel D. Palmer believed that deviations of the spinal column, referred to as *subluxations*, were the cause of practically all disease, and that chiropractic adjustments would be the cure. He used these adjustments to treat a variety of ailments including sciatica, migraine headaches, stomach complaints, epilepsy, and heart trouble. This type of philosophy was opposite to the practice of medicine; therefore it received very strong opposition from the medical establishment. In those days, chiropractors were jailed for practicing without a medical license, but their patients and followers persevered, bringing them into the light as healers and doctors.

Daniel D. Palmer did not live to see his discoveries accepted by the greater medical community; but his son, Dr. B.J. Palmer, carried on his father's passion and advanced the practice of chiropractic by getting it recognized as a licensed profession and establishing the Palmer School of Chiropractic, in Davenport, Iowa.

In the 1970's, Dr. Chang Ha Suh, a medical doctor working at the University of Colorado, conducted studies that provided extensive scientific research related to chiropractic. Since then, numerous important studies and research have added to the credibility of chiropractic. Today, chiropractic is the third largest primary health care profession in the United States. Many now consider chiropractic mainstream rather than alternative.

Frequently Asked Questions

What causes Scoliosis?

There are a few suggested causes; it can be hereditary, or caused by an injury. Some people believe uncorrected spinal damage from the birth process may be involved, while others suggest that encouraging children to walk too early, skipping the natural crawling stage, may be the culprit. The truth is that, for the most part, the cause is unknown.

Can Scoliosis be prevented?

Until now, there is no known way of preventing it from happening. Many people learn they have Scoliosis when seeing a chiropractic physician during a regular check-up, or going through a routine sports physical. There is a very simple test, called Adam's Test, which is part of the chiropractic exam protocol and as such, if there is a spinal abnormality, it is likely to be detected.

I've noticed that when I look in the mirror one of my shoulders is higher than the other, is that Scoliosis?

There are many other reasons to have one shoulder higher than the other. The best thing to do is to have your spine checked to determine the cause of your shoulder's being uneven. Doctors of chiropractic are trained to observe whether the structural alignment of the spinal column is normal or abnormal.

I heard that only girls get Scoliosis but my friend's brother, who is only 11 years old, has it. How can that be?

Scoliosis *can* affect both sexes, but more frequently girls between 8 years old and 18 years old.

Will adjustments hurt?

Not usually. Some patients experience mild soreness after being adjusted, but I find this to be rare. Most people feel better afterwards.

Are there side effects to being adjusted?

It is possible to feel tired afterward or even have some discomfort like a headache, but these minor side-effects tend to resolve within one or two days. I am used to seeing mostly positive side effects, like ache and pain going away, and the patient's telling me that, since they got adjusted, they experience an increase in energy, are sleeping better at night, and can feel an overall improvement of well-being afterward.

Still, it took about 77 years for all fifty states to establish licensing boards, and only a lawsuit finally prompted recognition and acceptance of the field by the American Medical Association in 1991.

Today, chiropractors are licensed in every state. There are over 50,000 practicing chiropractors in this country alone. Chiropractic continues to gain wide acceptance by the medical, legal, and patient communities through its long history of proven results. There is even an area of veterinary medicine that utilizes chiropractic techniques to treat animals.

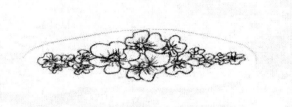

"If you think you *can't,* and think you *can't* long enough and strong enough, then you *can't* because you *won't*. But if you think *you can*, and you think *you can* long enough and strong enough, then you'll *try*; and in *trying*, you *will*."

"*Success* comes from hard work, long hours, being sincere, being honest with one's self, looking facts squarely and dealing with them frankly being open in relations with fellow men; thinking ten hours to percolate out one sane, sound, sensible idea in ten minutes. After all, *ideas* are what constitute the foundation upon which the superstructure of every success is built."

B.J. Palmer, Doctor of Chiropractic

Chiropractic Care in the Management of Scoliosis

Chiropractic adjustments to the spine have been proven to be one of the most helpful, holistic methods of managing and controlling the stiffness and pain that can accompany this condition.

Doctors of chiropractic are health care professionals trained to specifically address spinal problems. They emphasize *health maintenance* and *disease prevention* by teaching and encouraging proper nutrition, exercise, posture, and stress management, in addition to care of the spine and nervous system.

Besides keeping you under observation until you have reached bone maturity – which is the time when the spine as well as its curvature, stops growing, chiropractors use a very specific procedure called a "spinal adjustment." An adjustment is a specific movement applied to a joint to restore proper motion and function and eliminate nerve irritation. They use drugless therapies, like electrical stimulation, massage, heat, traction, and orthopedic supports as needed. They also pay close attention to lifestyle factors and make suggestions about diet, rest, exercise, and ergonomics, which often make a very positive impact on one's overall health. This integrated approach may help slow the progression of Scoliosis. Drugs or surgery are not part of the chiropractic philosophy, but if either *is* needed, a referral to the appropriate type of doctor will be made.

***

At present, the patient with Scoliosis has three choices when it comes to the traditional medical model:

1. Close observation (which is basically spine x-rays done every three to four months to keep track of changes in curvature).

2. Various bracing devices (which are indicated when the curve is between 20 and 40 degrees). Bracing doesn't correct the curve but it's supposed to prevent further progression. The brace is often worn 23 and ½ hours per day until skeletal maturity is reached.

3. Surgery is the third alternative, if the curve is more than 40 degrees. The most common surgeries include the insertion of Harrington's rods into the spine and the Dwyer procedure of wire cable and screws.

Besides possible internal obstruction due to compression, the use of external braces can affect the patient psychologically. On the other hand, progressive Scoliosis can seriously affect the lungs and the heart and choices become limited over time.

There are various complications that can happen with surgery such as cardiac arrest and spinal cord injury; postoperative problems can include infections, bony fusion, and failure of the mechanical devices intended to correct the problem.

Any form of surgery (cutting) is an invasive form of treatment and whenever possible it warrants a second opinion. Being a chiropractor I get to treat a lot of patients that tell me that, if they had been given a choice between back/neck surgery and chiropractic adjustments they would have chosen to try chiropractic first. Yet one must be open minded and realize there are times when surgery will save someone's life and a drug is needed for a specific illness.

**Leaves, like problems, waver
in falls's tempered winds.
Remember we must be like the
tree that rides out frustration's
storm; dormant, yet waiting
for spring's fresh thoughts.**

Danlar

How do I know I have stopped growing? I heard that once I stop growing, progression of my Scoliosis won't continue.

We stop growing at seventeen to eighteen years of age but if you want to make sure, ask your chiropractor. By looking at your X-rays, he or she can tell if you have reached bone maturity. Once you have stopped growing, rapid progression of your curve is unlikely to continue, even though slow progression of idiopathic curves can happen at 1 degree /year and is a recognized complication. This is the reason I feel strongly about **TESP** and chiropractic adjustments being an ongoing maintenance protocol through life.

My mother says that if I take calcium every day I will have strong bones. Is that all I have to do?

Calcium is important in your diet but there are other factors to be considered, like genetics, weight-bearing exercise, hormonal balance, diet, and the availability of bone building nutrients that help make calcium more absorbable – see pages 101-109.

I am 45 years old and I was told a year ago that I have mild Scoliosis. Should I worry about my spine?

Worrying is a strong term. I would rephrase that by encouraging you to follow the suggestions in this book. Take a look at the chapter on osteoporosis, and learn more about why you should maintain physically fit and healthy. Prevention is the key.

Do you have an easy suggestion of how I can check my child for Scoliosis?

Have your child in the standing position, preferably without a shirt and in their underpants, observe the following while standing behind him or her:

1. Is one shoulder higher than the other?
2. Do you notice one of the shoulder blades higher or more prominent than the other?
3. While standing straight with arms loosely at their side, is there more space between the arm and the body on one side?
4. Does it look like one hip is higher or more prominent than the other?
5. Still standing behind your child, ask him or her to bend over slowly and touch their toes, with head bent forward, until the spine is horizontal. Look at their back to see if one side appears higher than the other.

If you notice any problems or are at all unsure, a health-care professional, such as a chiropractor, should perform the evaluation. The critical time period for progression, which may be rapid, is between the ages of 12 and 16 years.

I am 16 years old. Once I stop growing do I still have to exercise?

Sherlock Holmes used to say after resolving a case, "Elementary, my dear Watson." To me this means, the answer is clear to see, dear friend.

If while growing up you recognize that **TESP** has made a positive impact in your life and has helped to address the curvature of your spine, my advice is that once you have "grown up" you should exercise two to three times a week to maintain a healthy you. This advice also goes towards continuing with chiropractic care, good eating habits, and a positive outlook in life, which you will hopefully be able to maintain throughout your future.

I was looking on the Internet and came across a few web sites on Scoliosis. They said to be aware of certain myths like; carrying a backpack will not cause Scoliosis. Is this true?

Wearing a backpack will not cause Scoliosis. But can aggravate it. If you are not wearing it over both shoulders, try this experiment in front of the mirror to see what happens:

Set the backpack strap over your lower shoulder for a few minutes; watch how hard it is to balance yourself, because the backpack keeps sliding off the lower shoulder. Now put the backpack over the high shoulder and notice how much more comfortable you are bending along with the curve. Do you really want to bend that way? This is the way most people with Scoliosis carry it because it is more comfortable, even though it's encouraging the spine to sustain the wrong curve. Some students carry backpacks with up to 40% of their body weight or more; imagine what that does to the spine, not to mention the backache that may cause. See page 17 for *Tips on Backpack Safety.*

Both my parents are constantly asking me, to sit straight. They say if I don't I'm going to start looking like my grandfather who walks all bent forward. Is that true? Can bad posture cause Scoliosis?

Without seeing your grandfather I am going to assume that his spinal curvature is only forward and if that is the case, than it is called Kyphosis, but if his spine also curves to one side then it is both Kyphosis and Scoliosis. Bad posture can aggravate and or cause those two conditions. Sitting in a slouched position or walking with our heads drooping forward can only add insult to injury by influencing the curvature of the spine and our health.

Hippocrates, the father of medicine, said "Look well to the spine for it is often the cause of sickness and disease."

The Importance of Good Posture

Dr. Roger Sperry, 1998 Nobel Peace Prize winner for brain research, said "With poor posture, only 10% of the brain's energy output is used for thinking, metabolism and healing the body from illness."

Mood can affect posture as well as posture can affect our mood. When we are sad we tend to round our backs with the shoulders slouching and our head hanging forward. Even the lips tend to go down on the corners. Through my years of practice I've had a few young patients tell me that once they started walking with their shoulders back and sitting up straight, life in general seemed to have gotten better and they had more friends.

Some obvious causes of bad posture: Scoliosis; constant injuries; poor sleep support (mattress); injury to muscles, tendons, or bones; emotional problems; stress; job (improper ergonomic computer set up); excessive weight; improper nutrition; or visual problems. Unless there is a structural deformity or disease, the chances for correction or improvement are good. My niece is the perfect example of a case history involving a Kyphotic spine, which was corrected by postural awareness.

I was visiting my sister-in-law Vicki, during a school break from Chiropractic College West, and she asked me what could be done to help her daughter Erin. She was concerned with Erin's severe forward curvature of the spine. I told her I would definitely adjust Erin that day to help with some of the backache, but I believed there wasn't much more that could be done. Erin was twenty years old, and as such she had reached full skeletal maturity. I couldn't even *imagine* anything that could help her spine to go straight.

Erin had a petite frame and over the years had gotten used to maintaining her shoulders forward as if to hide her breasts. I was in my second year of practice when I heard that upon finishing college Erin had gone to Japan to teach English to young children. One year later she decided to remain a second year teaching in Japan. Two years went by and I got a chance to see Erin again when she decided to return to the USA and make her home in Portland, Oregon.

My first question upon seeing her was, "Erin your back is straight! Did you have back surgery?"

Her answer caught me by surprise. "In Japan, posture is very important. I had to sit and stand straight in front of my class if I was going to receive their respect. In the beginning, it was very painful and definitely not easy to bring my shoulders back and maintain an erect posture, but I did it day after day until it became a habit."

The results were impressive. She had proven to me that posture was very important, and that with perseverance nothing is impossible. Erin had done it for the love of teaching; what might motivate you?

Bad posture can also affect our breathing!

Remain seated, bend forward with your back arched and let your head hang down.
Hold about 3 minutes and take notice of your breathing, then try to take a deep breath while still holding the same seated position.
Now, straighten up your back, bring your shoulders up and chest out, level your head above the shoulders. Pay attention to breathing, notice how much easier it is to fill your lungs with air. Take a deep breath and enjoy the oxygen you are bringing into the lungs and brain. Give thanks for the simple blessing of breathing.

Posture can also be affected by many other factors besides emotion or personal neglect, like genetics, injuries, aging, deformities, or simply wanting to "fit" into the present society, which can have a negative effect in the way we carry ourselves. Sometimes girls will try to hide their breasts by bending forward and the boys will do the same just because everybody else does it. If correction starts while still young, then posture issues are easier to address.

By becoming aware of how we sit and stand we can make an instant change to postural distortion. On the first visit to my office, if a young patient sits slouching while I am taking a history of their present complaint I excuse myself from the room. Once back in the exam room, I ask if they mind holding the position they are presently using because I need to take a side picture of their back with my automatic camera. Next, I invite them to sit straight and hold their shoulders back for the next photograph. After that, I show them both pictures.

The results have been very encouraging and for the most part patients are open to having a family member remind them to sit straight. Hopefully when they stop growing, these young patients will have attained a natural, good posture. The goal is prevention. Nobody wants to look like the typical "old folks" when we get older.

"Most of the shadows of this life are caused by our standing in our own sunshine."

Ralph Waldo Emerson

Tips on Backpack Safety

- **Distribute the weight evenly.** Put the heavier items on the bottom to keep the weight off your shoulders and help you maintain better posture.

- **Wear both shoulder straps unless your pack is designed for use on one shoulder.** Carrying a heavy backpack using one strap can shift weight to one side which can lead to neck and muscles spasms, low back pain, and walking improperly.

- **Choose backpacks that have heavily padded shoulder straps.** Non-padded straps dig into the shoulders causing pain due to compressional loading of the acromio-clavicular joints in the shoulder and stress on the trapezius muscles.

- **Choose a backpack that has a lumbar cushion.** The lumbar cushion will redistribute weight to the lower extremities, creating a fulcrum (a pivot) that facilitates an upright standing position.

The Congress of Chiropractic State Associations and the International Chiropractic Pediatric Association are recommending the "AirPack Backpack" designed by Core Products, which seems to provide revolutionary comfort and support by reducing stress on the shoulders and back by 80% and lightening the effective load by 50%. Its ergonomic design combines wider shoulder straps and an inflatable lumbar cushion which, when properly positioned, redistributes the weight from the shoulders to the hips promoting a healthier upright standing posture.

YOUR WEIGHT	RECOMENDED PACK WEIGHT
50 lbs	5 to 7.5 lbs
80 lbs	8 to 12 lbs
100 lbs	10 to 15 lbs
130 lbs	13 to 19.5 lbs
150 lbs	15 to 17.5 lbs

* Recommended pack weight is equal to 10-15% of bodyweight.

Buying a backpack is no different than buying a pair of shoes, consideration for your back should be addressed as well since it is working hard at keeping you up!

TESP (The Esagui Scoliosis Protocol)

Before beginning *TESP*, one must understand that our bodies work at different levels of efficiency which can be influenced by two main factors; age and present health status. Most of all, we must remember that we can never compare ourselves to another being, some of us heal faster while others need more patience and need to be more proactive. Set goals that make sense and apply to you.

Check with your chiropractic physician before beginning *TESP* to make sure the exercises are appropriate for you and your specific needs. If you experience recurring, sharp, or shooting pain, stop and report back to your chiropractor. You may need to modify the exercises to fit your personal needs.

Ask your doctor to show you your "full spine X-ray" and to give you a mini anatomy/skeletal lesson so that you can better understand the structure and biomechanics of what's involved. This will give you a visual idea as to what you are working with and what you are striving to accomplish.

For best results perform *TESP* on a daily basis, your spine and wellbeing depend on it.

Take one day at a time and look forward to the next day.

Good health is not a gift. It has to be cultivated and cared for.

Exercising is synonymous with loosing fat, gaining muscle tone, and improving mental health.

Fitness = Health

"There is no drug in current or prospective use that holds as much promise for sustained health as a lifetime program of physical exercise," says Dr. Walter M. Bortz II in the *Journal of the American Medical Association.*

Starting *TESP*

Here are some suggestions:

Pick a day when you have forty-five minutes to an hour free to go over *TESP* in this book and become familiar with each move. Start with two to three exercises per day and keep adding a new one each day. Another idea is getting a friend or family member to be your partner in health. Make a pact to encourage each other. Ask this person to give you a friendly reminder every day.

Besides chiropractic adjustments to the spine, exercise is a very important part of the chiropractic life-style. After you get your spine adjusted, staying active on a daily basis will reinforce muscles, ligaments, and discs, and help maintain spinal alignment. If you know that your curvature is twenty degrees or more, you should be doing *TESP* two times per day.

What to wear

Wear what feels comfortable and allows for easy movement. The least you wear the more freedom of movement you'll have. This is the reason I prefer to do my daily *TESP* workout when I get up in the morning, naked. If one were comfortable, doing so, this might be the best method!

Where to do *TESP*

Anywhere you like, since it has to fit your daily routine. Are you going to school or to work? Are you home for the summer or traveling?

I like to start my day by working out as soon as I get up in the morning. It's like welcoming the day ahead where, no matter what happens, it's going to be awesome.

I sit up in bed and begin with the neck exercises. The majority of the time, I still have my eyes closed. I also perform the floor exercises in the bedroom. For the standing exercises I use the bathroom, which has a great countertop for the legs work out. I keep track of my posture in the mirror above the countertop. A hot shower followed by breakfast is my reward, and I start the day feeling energized.

What you need to invest in:

1. Yourself.
2. Chiropractic way of life and spinal adjustments.
3. A healthy diet. (Check page 69 for Healthy Hints)
4. If you don't have a comfortable carpet in your bedroom, get a mat. (A non-slip mat is recommended.)
5. Get two three to five pound weights. Small weights are inexpensive and easy to store under your bed.
6. Maintain a healthy outlook on life.

Even if you have not had recent surgery or any muscle or joint problems, consult your chiropractor before starting *TESP* or any other type of exercise program. He or she will evaluate your condition and properly advise the course of action you need to follow.

Always stretch slowly. Don't worry how far you can stretch; before you know it, limberness will be your end result.

Don't go beyond your limits; if it becomes painful, you are over stretching.

It shouldn't take more than forty minutes each morning to do *TESP*

Go to bed forty minutes earlier if you need that extra time to sleep. You don't want to be exercising while wishing you were still sleeping.

Besides helping with curvature of the spine, *TESP* is a gentle, easy way of helping with stress, muscle tension, increasing flexibility, joint mobility, and improving heart health. The list of health benefits from exercise is quite long. To put it simply, our bodies are made to move and they thrive on it.

I will not address what muscles are being involved with each movement; the main focus of *TESP* is where in the spine you should be feeling its effect.

TESP works specially to extend the spine, increase the elasticity of the muscles, and improve the flexibility of joints. Chiropractic adjustments and *TESP* compliment each other as they are founded on the philosophy that a healthy spine creates balance and clears the nervous system.

Before starting *TESP* take your time to look over each picture. I put *TESP* together in the order I found it to be most practical to follow, but you should still see your chiropractor before starting this program since every spine is slightly different. If you get discomfort or pain from performing *TESP*, I encourage you to stop and see your doctor. To reduce the potential for injury, *TESP* should be performed under the guidance of your doctor.

Personalizing TESP for *Your* Spine

Use this page when in doubt as to which side you need to be bending. Seeing your X-ray with your chiropractor can be very beneficial since you will get advice and a better idea as to which is your high side of the curve. You always want to go <u>against the curve</u> as shown below.

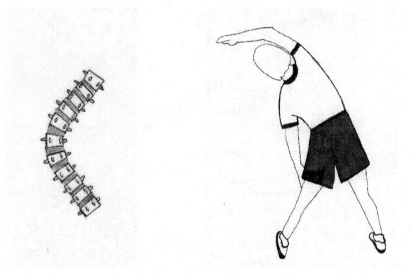

If the curve is to the left, **(the high side)** exercises are performed to the left side, moving your spine <u>against the curve.</u>

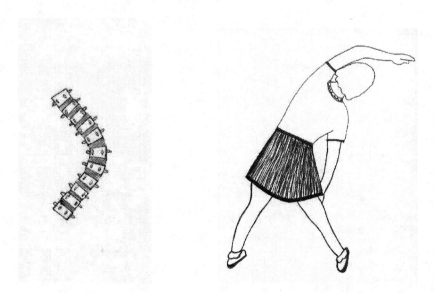

If the curve is to the right, **(the high side)** exercises are performed to the right side, moving your spine <u>against the curve</u>.

Imagine!

Think
of yourself
as a unique and
perhaps exotic plant growing in the
center of a beautiful Caribbean island.

You
    have
      been
        growing
          all these years
            just ever so slightly
            off to the side,
            going along
              with the warm
                yet cooling ocean
                  breeze for so long
                    that you can't even imagine
                      what it must be like to stand straight.

Would you like to be flexible in both directions and have an all around ocean view?

Imagine the change first.
Now, let's do something about it!
Follow me to *TESP*!

Neck Flexion and Extension (Sitting position)

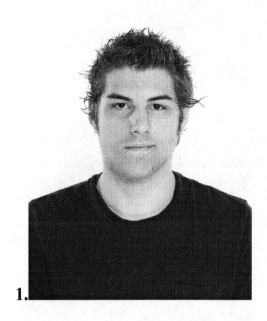

1.

Sit erect with hands to the side.

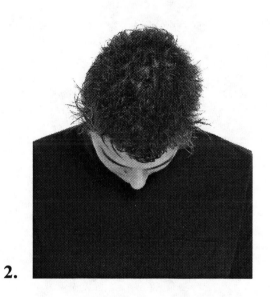

2.

Slowly, bring your head forward into flexion. (Exhale during this motion) **You should feel a slight stretching of the back-of-neck muscles and upper back muscles.**

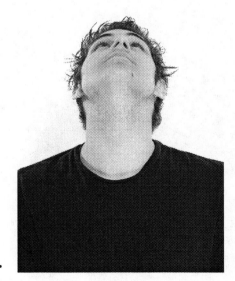

3.

Extend head back gently. (Inhale during this motion) **You should feel the front-of-neck muscles stretching. Repeat flexion and extension 10 times, slowly.**

Head Roll (Remain seated)

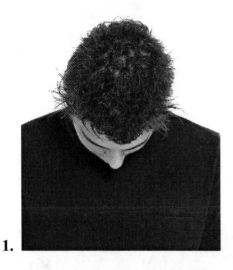

1.

Slowly bring chin to chest.
(Feel the stretch in back of your
neck and upper back)

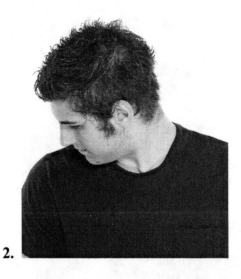

2.

**Rotate head gently to the right side.
Take your time with this up motion.**
(You should feel the left neck muscles
being stretched)

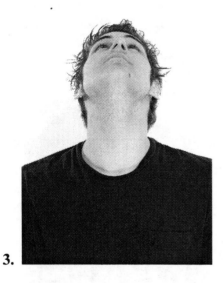

3.

**Continue to rotate until head
is extended back comfortably.**
(Feel the stretch in the front of
your neck)

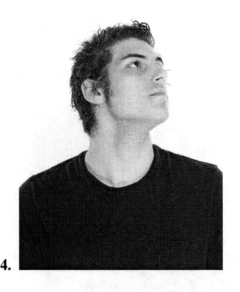

4.

**Gently rotate head to the left,
finishing clockwise rotation.**
(Feel the stretch on your right
side of your neck)

Perform *Head Roll* 5 times clockwise and 5 times counterclockwise.

Seated Wing Stretch (Remain seated)

- **TESP** should be performed slowly and smoothly so that you can get maximum benefit.
- Stretch to where you feel a slight easy stretch in your mid and upper back. If it becomes painful, you are over stretching.
- Do not jerk or bounce from one position to another.
- Always breath slowly and rhythmically.

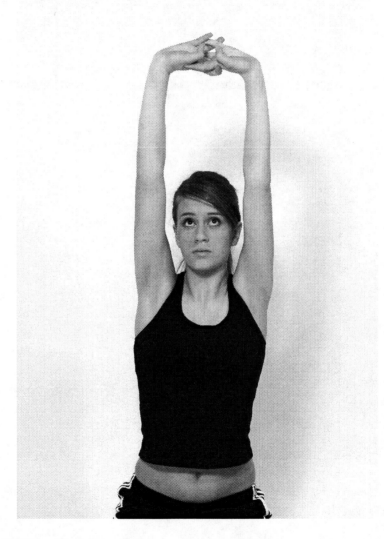

1. **Take a deep breath.**
2. **Stretch arms up to the ceiling, keeping your back erect.**
3. **Hold 5 seconds.** (Feel it in your mid and upper back)
4. **Exhale while you bring arms down to the sides of your body.**
5. **Do once.**

Second Wing Stretch (Standing)

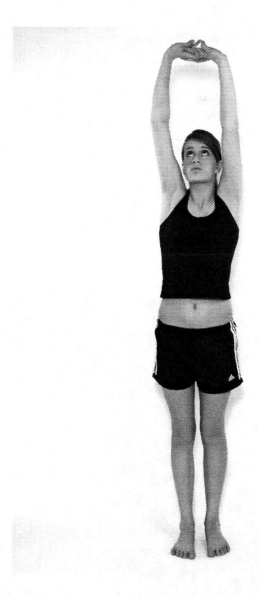

1. **Take a deep breath as you stretch arms up to the ceiling and keeping your back erect.** (Feel your spine elongate)
2. **Hold 5 seconds.**
3. **Exhale while you bring arms down to the sides of your body.**
4. **Do once.**

You will notice that this second stretch feels even better than the first, that's because now you can feel your muscles stretching easier along with the spine. You are now ready to ***Welcome the New Day.***

Welcome the New Day

• You should never *Welcome the New Day* in a hurry. Feel the joy of waking up to a new start of positive thoughts and learning experiences. Take your time! It is a new day! Welcome it with a smile.

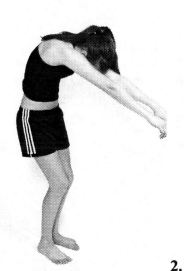

1.
Bend knees slightly.
Bring arms together.
Bend head forward.

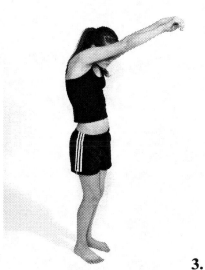

2.
Come up slowly.
Bring head up with arms.
Stretch arms up straight.

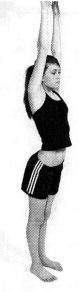

3.
Reach for the sky.

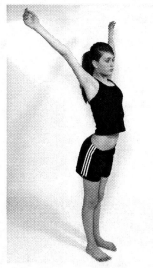

4.
Gently open arms as if hugging the world.
(Feel it across your upper back)

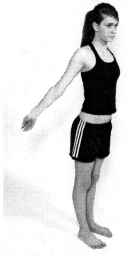

5.
Bring chest out.
(Feel it across your upper and mid back, take a deep breath)

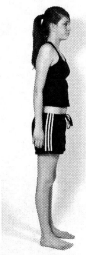

6.
Bring arms down.
(Exhale)

Repeat 10 times.

Push Up 101

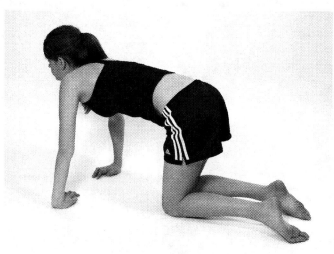

1. **Kneel as pictured.**
2. **Keep your head up and your back straight.** (Feel it in back of your neck)
3. **Place hands facing in under shoulder level.**
4. **Pull in your belly button and abdominal muscles.**

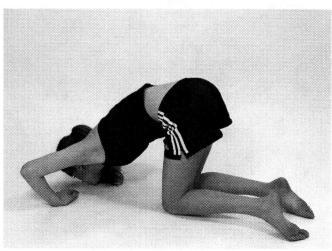

5. **Allow upper body to lower slowly while keeping spine straight and head up.**
6. **"Kiss" the floor.**
   (Feel the stretch in your lower neck, and mid upper back, particularly between the shoulder blades)
7. **Hold 3 seconds.**

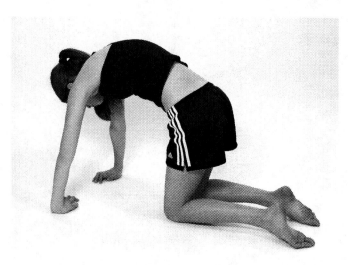

8. **Slowly arch your entire spine as you bring the pelvis forward.**
9. **Keep chin to chest while keeping abdominal muscles tight.**
10. **Hold position 3 seconds.**

Repeat "Push Up 101" 10 times.

Modified Push Up 101

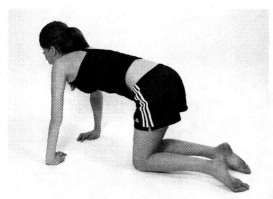

1. Return to kneeling position with your head up, as in *Push Up 101*.

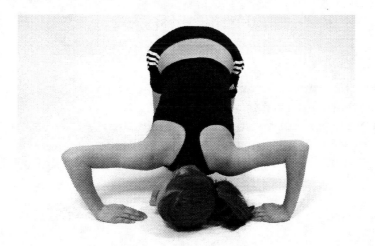

2. Allow upper body to drop slowly with head turned to the right side, while placing the left ear to the floor. Hold 3 seconds. (Feel it between your shoulder blades)

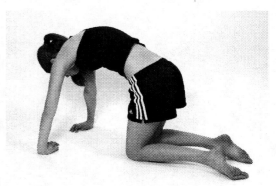

3. Slowly arch entire spine as you bring the pelvis forward. Keep chin to chest while keeping abdominal muscles tight as in *Push Up 101*. Hold 2-3 seconds.

Repeat *Modified Push Up 101*, 5 times to the <u>right</u> side and 5 times to the <u>left</u> side.

Cat Stretch

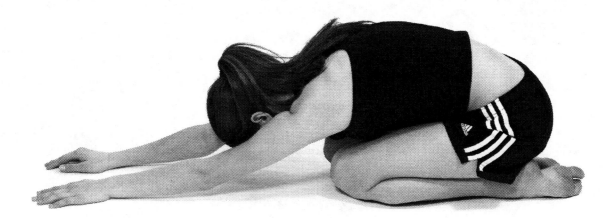

1. **Remain on your knees and sit on your heels** (as picture).
2. **Reach gently forward in a straight line.**
3. **Stretch the spine as you reach your arms forward. Hold for 10 seconds.**
4. **Breathe slowly and rhythmically, maintain the position while you inhale and exhale.** (Notice your spine slowly stretching each time you exhale)
5. **Do once.**

Stretch and Grow

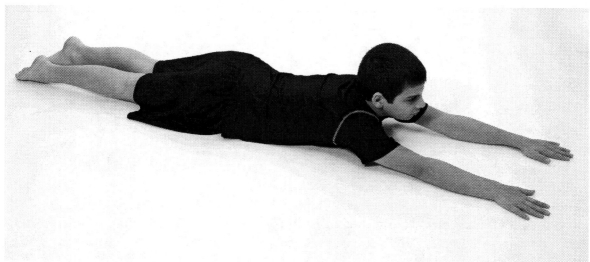

1. **Lay flat on the floor keeping your head up and stretch arms forward.**
2. **Keep your head up. Stretch legs out with pointed toes and tighten buttocks while pressing the pelvis to the floor. Hold for 5 seconds.** (Feel it in back of your neck and back) **Do once.**

Against the Rainbow (The high side of the curve)

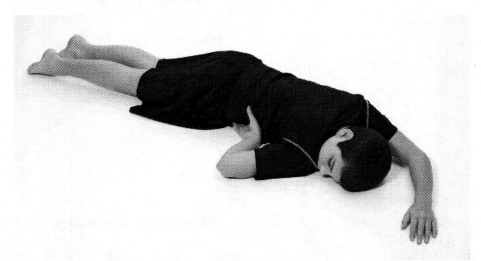

1. **Remain on your stomach and reach up as high as you can with the left hand.** (If your spinal curve is to the right you will need to bend to the right side, **(against the curve)** as the model is in this picture.
2. **Turn your head to the right as it is in this case, positioning the right hand on your waist.** (Feel the stretch on your whole left side)
3. **Hold for 5 seconds. Do once.**

Swimming

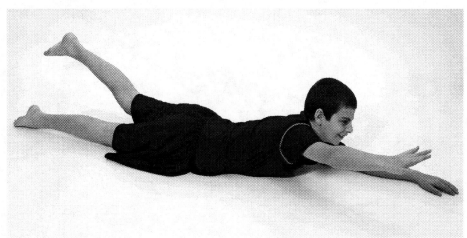

1. **Remain flat on the floor. Keep head up.**
2. **Raise one hand and opposite leg about 6 inches off the floor.**
3. **Hold 3 seconds. (Feel it through your back and neck)**
4. **Alternate sides 5 times.**

– If you have no **Scoliosis** and are doing **TESP** to stay fit, maintain a healthy spine, and muscle tone, please perform *Side Scissors, Knee to Elbow* and *Mermaid Lift* on both sides.

– If your curve is to the left side you should be lying down on your right side. Remember, you want to go against the curve. When not sure, check **Personalizing TESP for your spine.** (Page 21)

Side Scissors (Going against the curve)

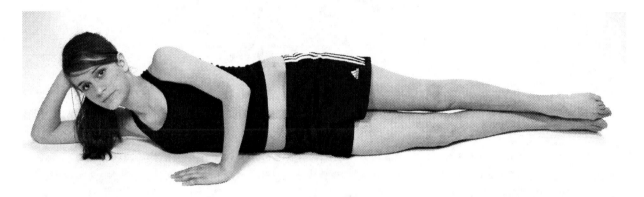

1. **Lay down on "your" side with hand and elbow positioned to stabilize the body.**
2. **Take a full breathe, exhale and relax.**

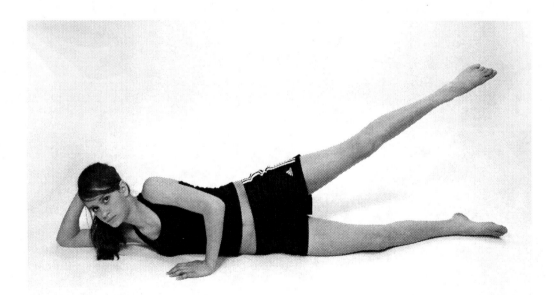

3. **Slowly raise your upper leg as high as you can. Don't use momentum to bring leg up. Use your upper arm and hand to help you keep your back and pelvis straight.**
4. **Gently lower your leg to starting position, but don't allow your leg to rest when it comes down. Try to keep the movement smooth.** (Feel it on your lower back, around your waist)
5. **Repeat same side 10 times.**

Knee to Elbow (Going against the curve)

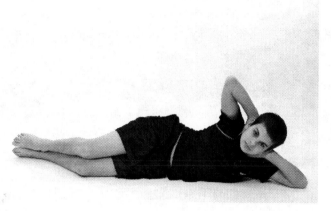

1. Remain on "your" side.
2. Keep knees slightly bent.
3. Place both hands behind your head.
4. Use the elbow on the floor for support.

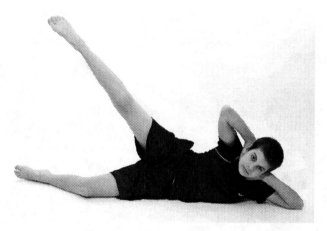

5. Raise your top leg straight up, slowly.
6. Keep your back straight and tighten up your abdominal muscles.

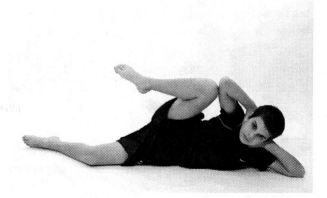

7. Bend your knee and bring it towards you to meet your elbow. (Feel the movement on your lower back and around your waist)
8. Hold position 3 seconds. Don't bring your leg down to rest until you have repeated knee to elbow contraction 10 times.

Mermaid Lift (Going against the curve)

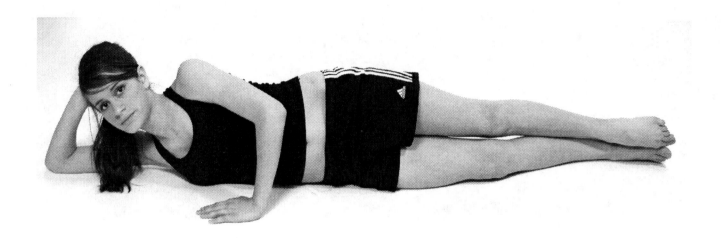

1. Remain on "your" side.
2. Extend both your legs straight out.

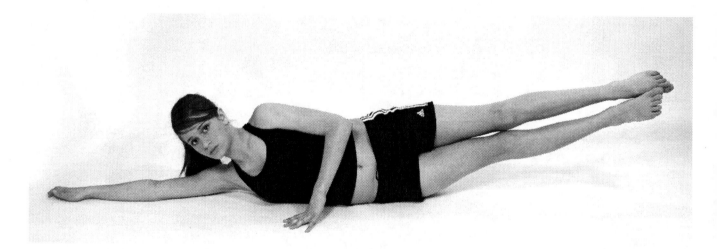

3. Stretch arm out and use your upper arm and hand to help you keep the upper body elevated.
4. Raise both legs off the floor as high as you can while you try your best to raise the upper body as well.
5. Hold yourself up for 5 seconds. (This movement will be felt throughout your lower back)
6. Repeat 5 times.

- While you are performing **TESP** on your back, it is very important to use the following two stretches to help you cope with possible discomfort to your spine. You must realize that when you are working on reversing the curvature it can be very demanding on the spine and the muscles.
- *Knees to Chest* and *Stretch and Grow II* are very relaxing and refreshing to the spine. Feel free to use these two stretches any time you feel like resting your back from prolonged seating or standing.

Knees to Chest

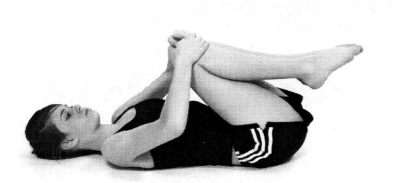

1. **Lying on your back, bring both your knees up.**
2. **Use hands to gently hold knees to your abdomen.**
3. **Keep your back flat, head down, and relax neck.**
4. **Hold knees up 3 seconds.** (Feel your spine opening and stretching against the floor)
5. **Do once.**

Stretch and Grow II

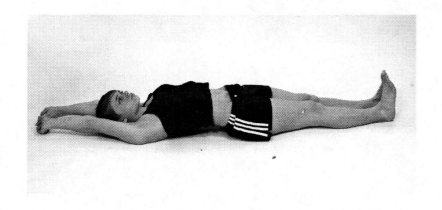

1. **Remain on your back.**
2. **Extend your arms above your head.**
3. **With hands together, stretch spine against the floor, by bringing hips slightly up to help press the lower back into the floor. Bring your toes up gently.**
4. **Maintain your back flat, against the floor**
5. **Hold 5 seconds.**
6. **Do once.**

The ABS Curl

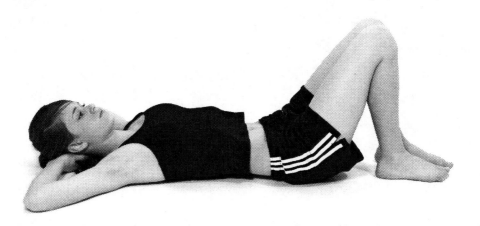

1. **Remain flat on your back. Bend your knees and keep the feet flat on the floor.**
2. **Support neck with fingers. Relax.**

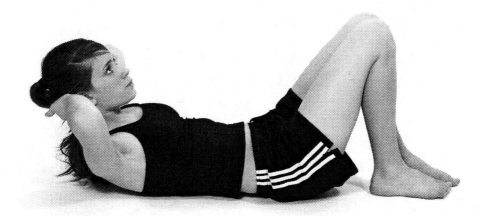

3. **Don't pull your head up with your hands. Your fingers are only there to support the weight of your head. Relax the neck.**
4. **Use the abdominal muscles to bring you up.**
5. **Keep your lower back as if glued flat to the floor.** (You are working out your abdominal muscles but you are also stretching your spine)
6. **Maintain a relaxed neck. Hold 3 seconds.**
7. **Repeat 10 times. Relax.**

Perform ***Stretch and Grow*** and ***Knees to Chest*** before continuing with ***TESP***.

Opposite Elbow to Knee

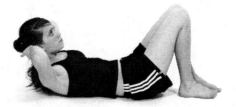

1. Remain flat on your back. Put your hands behind the neck as previously to support your neck.

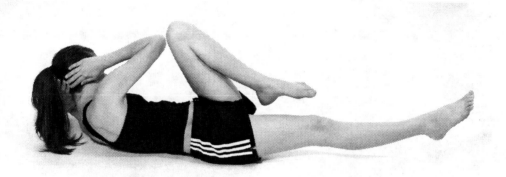

2. Extend one leg out and bring the opposite knee up to meet the opposing elbow. Hold for two counts. Only upper body should twist. Exhale as you come to center, inhale while switching sides. (Feel it through your spine, and the back and front trunk muscles)

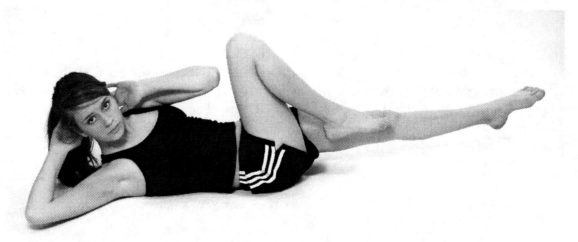

3. Repeat 10 times to each side in a smooth controlled motion.

• Make sure you keep the lower back flat and that your upper body twists along with the shoulders involved on the same side as you come up to meet the opposite knee.

When needed perform *Stretch and Grow* and *Knees to Chest* before continuing with *TESP*.

Scissors

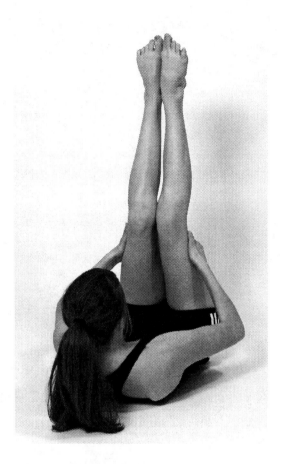 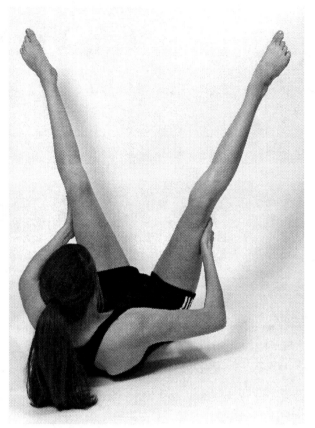

1. **Remain on your back.**
2. **Bring legs straight up, perpendicular to your body** (knees unlocked).
3. **Use abdominal muscles to help you sustain your head and upper back up.**

4. **Use hands to grasp the back of the knees.**
5. **Maintain lower back flat as you open and close legs.** (Feel it between mid and lower back)
6. **Repeat 10 times.**

- Don't forget to rest your back with *Stretch and Grow* and *Knees to Chest* when you need to relax the spine.

The Bridge (For the upper back)

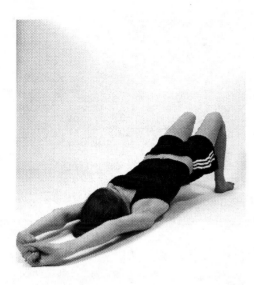

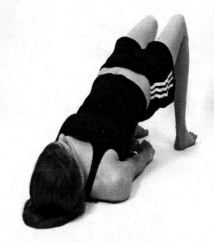

1. Keep knees bent, and feet flat on the floor.
2. Slowly bring pelvis up while retaining upper back flat on the ground.
3. Bring arms up into a stretch.
4. Hold 3 seconds.

5. Bring arms to side of body, and tuck them in straight along the spine. Keep pelvis up.
6. Hold 3 seconds.

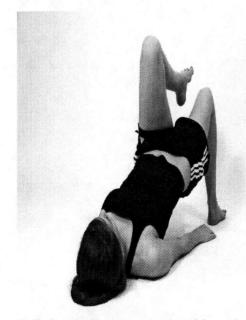

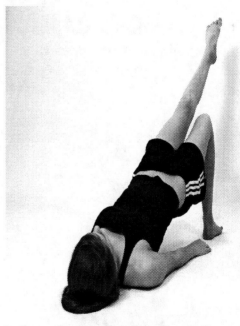

7. Relax both arms to the sides of your body.
8. Keeping your pelvis up bring your left knee up towards your abdomen.

9. Stretch out the left leg as high as you can.
10. Hold position 5 seconds.
11. Repeat 10 times with each leg.

Crisscross

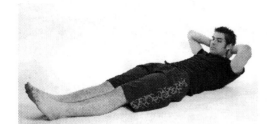

1. **Keep your lower back flat against the floor and bring your head up supported by your hands.**

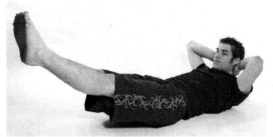

2. **Use abdominal muscles to keep your legs up.** (Feel it on the abdominal muscles, while making sure that your lower back is comfortable against the floor)

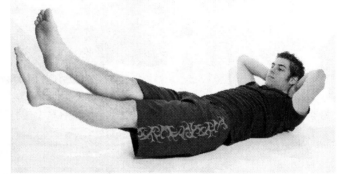

3. **Crisscross your legs back and forth.**
4. **Don't rest your feet on each other.**
5. **Crisscross works on the abdominal muscles.**

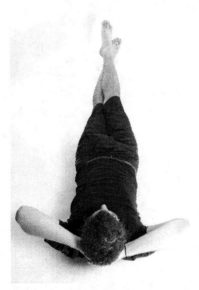

6. **Repeat 10 times with each leg.**

• After Crisscross relax your back with *Stretch and Grow* and *Knees to Chest.* Use those two stretches whenever you feel your spine needs a rest.

Roll Up and Curl

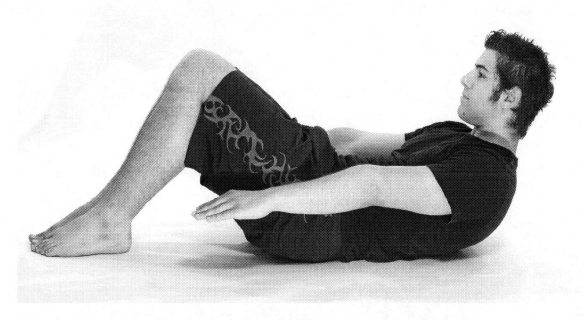

1. Keep feet and low back flat on the floor with knees bent.
2. Use your upper back and abdominal muscles instead of your hands to sustain your head up in position. Try to keep head flexed forward and chin in, if possible.
3. Curl upper body towards pelvis with both arms parallel to your body.
4. Keep your mid and lower back flat against the floor while pulling your upper back upwards.
5. Hold position 3 seconds. (Feel it in the lower and mid back)
6. Do once.

"I am determined to be the best I can be. I will exercise everyday and follow a healthy life-style everyday. Someday I will be a Marine."

Stephen (13 years old) 2008

Sit Up I

For the next three **TESP** sit ups, the most important thing to remember is to keep your back erect with the head up, chest out and shoulders straight. Use your arms to support and maintain your back straight. If done correctly you will feel the effect throughout your spine, particularly the mid and upper back.

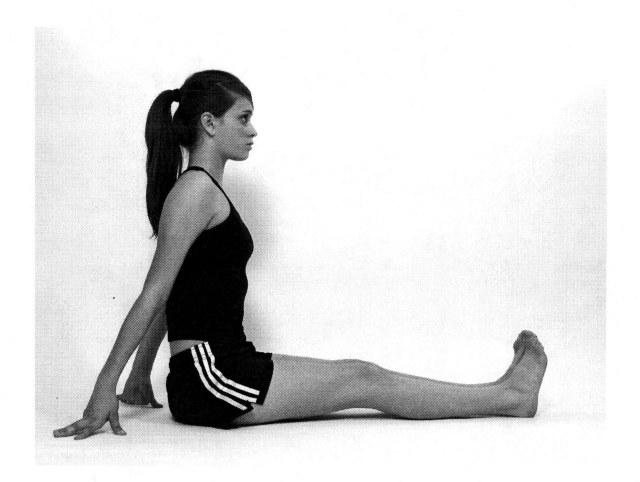

1. **Sit with both your legs straight feet together and toes up.**
2. **Support your back with both arms to keep it straight** (as pictured).
3. **Hold 2-3 seconds. Do once.**

Sit Up II

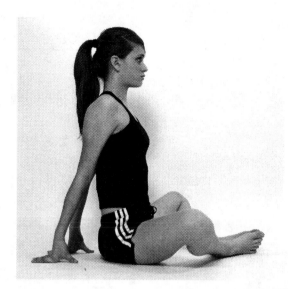

1. Remaining seated with your spine erect bring the feet together towards you.
2. Take a full breath, exhale and relax. Hold 2-3 seconds. Do once.

Sit Up III

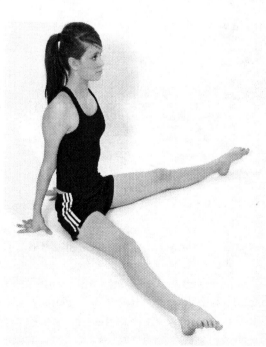

1. Remain seated and open your legs as wide as you can using arms to support and keep the spine straight.
2. Take a full breath, exhale, and relax. Hold 2-3 seconds. Do once.

Twist and Turn I

1. Do not force your body to twist.
2. Use inhalation to stretch and exhalation for rotating your hip and shoulders along with gentle twisting.
3. Try to maintain the buttocks from lifting off the floor.
4. Do your best to keep your back straight like you did in the previous *Sit Ups.*

Twist and Turn I and *II* will help you to keep the spine flexible by retaining side-to-side mobility.

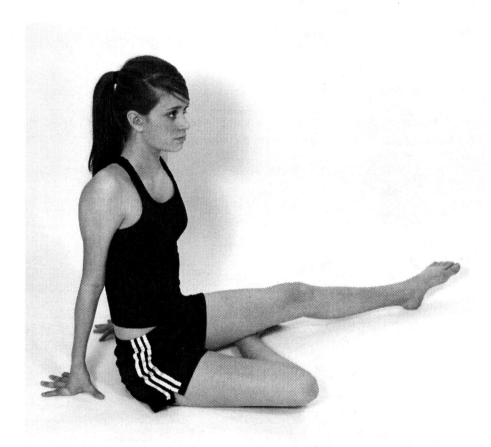

1. Remain seated with your back straight as you bend the right knee.

• Notice how the model is keeping her back straight throughout *TESP* but in the next picture she is leaning back rather than twisting up, because her right hand is too far away from her back. If you lean back you will loose the benefits of lateral stretching your spine, back muscles and hips.

Twist and Turn I (Cont.)

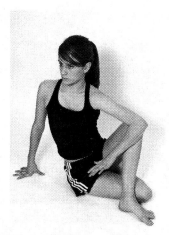

(The model's back is not straight because she is leaning instead of twisting)

2. Lift your left foot and put it on the floor outside the right thigh.
3. Position your right hand flat on the floor close to your back. (The model has her hand too far away from the body causing her to lean back, the hand should be closer to the hip bearing little or no weight)
4. Bring your left arm over your left leg and push gently against the left knee.
5. Hold 5 seconds. Breathe deep and lift through your rib cage to lengthen your spine. Exhale.
6. Do once.

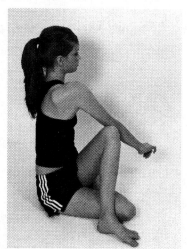

(The model is twisting correctly in this picture. Notice her straight spine)

1. Keep legs in the same position as before and gently twist your torso to the left side as you bring both your arms also to the left side.
2. Position your left hand flat on the floor close to your back and use your right arm to gently push against the left knee towards your body. Hold 5 seconds.
3. Breathe deep and exhale as before. Do once.

Twist and Turn II

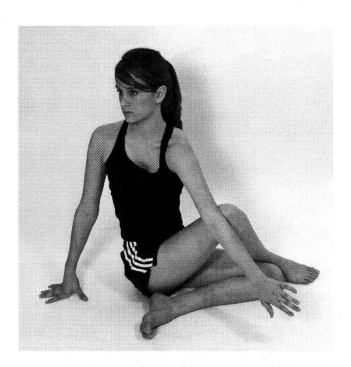

1. **Lift your right foot and put it flat on the floor outside the left thigh.**
2. **Position your right hand flat on the floor close to your back.**
3. **Bring your left arm over your left leg and push gently against the right knee. Hold 5 seconds.**
4. **Breathe deep and lift through your rib cage to lengthen your spine.**
5. **Exhale. Do once and then repeat to the left as shown in the picture below.**

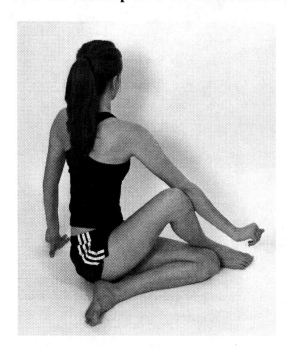

Getting Up (Full spine stretch)

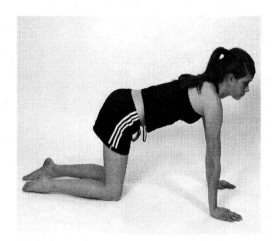

1. Start while kneeling as shown.
2. Keep head up and hands flat on the floor.

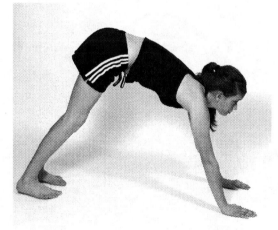

3. Raise your hips as high as possible.
4. Keep your head up.
5. Hold 2 seconds.

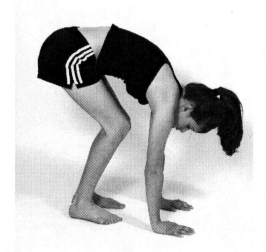

6. Keep knees slightly bent, as you take one or two steps forward, towards your hands.
7. When comfortable start bringing your hands towards your ankles.

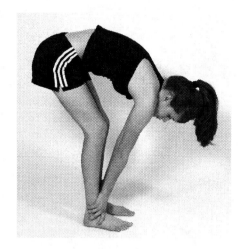

8. Hold this position with your hands at the ankles.
9. Keep your knees slightly bent.
10. Let your body relax for 2-3 seconds.

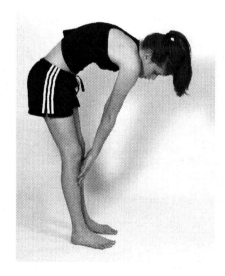

11. Come up slowly until you are standing up straight.

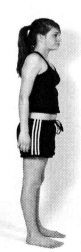

12. Inhale deeply. Exhale.

Runner's Start (Full spine stretch)

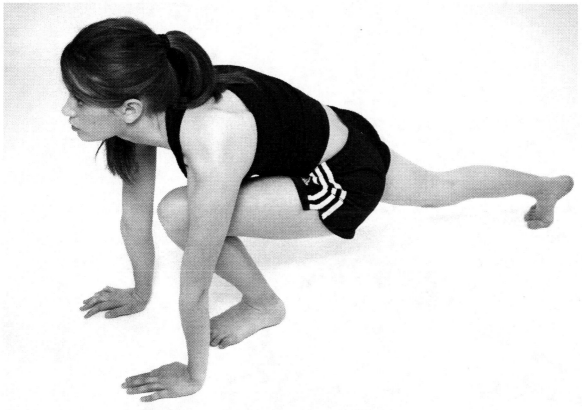

1. **From position "all-fours" set your hands facing forwards**
2. **Bring hips forward and lift your head upward into extension.**
3. **Bend left leg into a lunge with knee touching chest.**
4. **Stretch out your right leg without bending the knee.**
5. **Use hands to balance.**
6. **Keep your head in alignment with the spine.**
7. **Hold position for 5 seconds.** (Feel the stretch from back of your neck to the end of your lower spine)
8. **Repeat 2 times with each leg.**

"Although your spine may not be straight, don't worry. It's not too late.
Hang on to your hope. Think positive thoughts. You know you can help.
Give it all you've got!"

Molly (13 years old) 2006

Runner's Reach

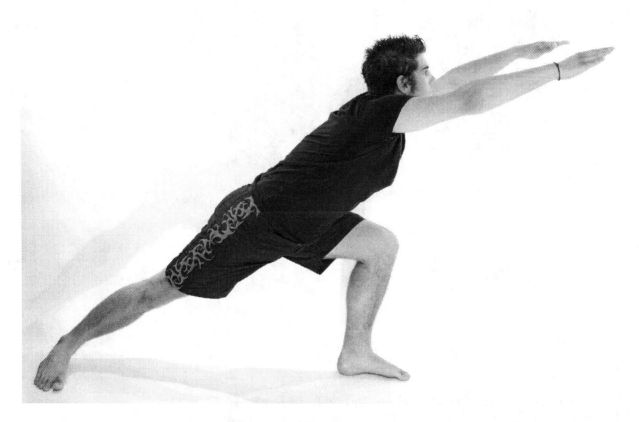

1. **Turn your upper body to the left side, facing the left knee bent.**
2. **Stretch out the right leg with the right foot turned at 90 degrees to the right.**
3. **Stretch both arms over your left knee and see how far you can gently stretch your spine by reaching out.** (Feel it throughout your spine)
4. **Hold 5 seconds.**
5. **Repeat *Runner's Reach* to the right side.**

"Believe in yourself and don't give up on your hopes and dreams.
Surround yourself with the eagles and fly along with them."

Jacob (16 years old) 2007

Reinforcing your Balance

For ***Tap your Foot,*** you will need a chair or something of similar height. I use the side of the bathtub instead of a chair because I do the following in the bathroom where I take advantage of the counter, which is the perfect height for ***Legs Up*** and the mirror is right above it.

What room you use should be whichever is practical for you. As one patient told me, his house is small but since his son moved out, he and his wife have turned their son's bedroom into their "personal gym and art studio."

Tap your Foot for Balance

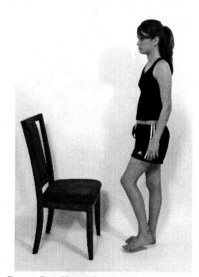 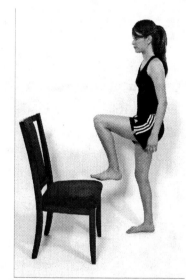

1. **Stand tall and erect.**
2. **Keep shoulders back and your head straight.**

3. **Hold abdomen in as you lift your left leg to barely touch the chair.**
4. **Repeat 10 times with each foot.**

"I saw the angel in the marble and carved until I set it free."

Michelangelo

The Balancing Act

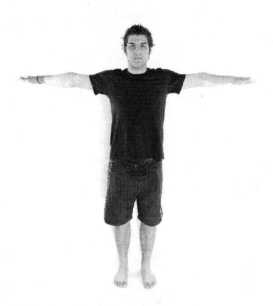

1. Facing the mirror open your arms.

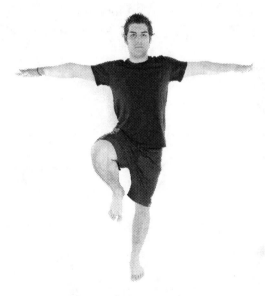

2. Lift your right foot.

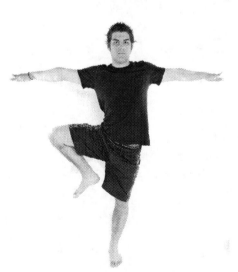

3. Keep right knee bent, and bring it
to the side. Use arms out for balance.

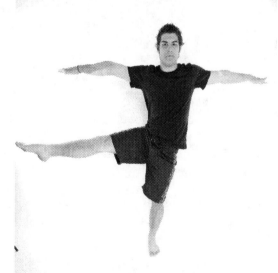

4. Stretch leg out slowly. Keep balance.
Repeat on the other side.

Legs Up, Phase I (In front of the mirror)

(Addresses the spine and the muscles of the back, the legs and hips)

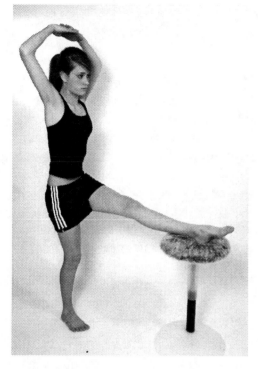

In this picture the model is using an unwavering stool to help her keep her leg up. Make sure what you use is stable.

1. **Place your left foot up on a secure support of some kind,** (counter top, table, chair) **height should be to your comfort.**
2. **Keep your back and both your legs straight.**
3. <u>**Bend your elbows**</u> **and bring your hands together above your head.**
4. **Inhale deeply and exhale while stretching your spine upwards.**
5. **Hold position 5 seconds. Do once.**

6. **Keep prior position with your back upright and left leg extended.** (Use mirror to help confirm your posture).
7. <u>**Stretch arms up,**</u> **holding hands together above your head.**
8. **Inhale deeply and exhale while stretching your spine upwards.**
9. **Hold position 5 seconds. Do once.**

Legs Up Phase II

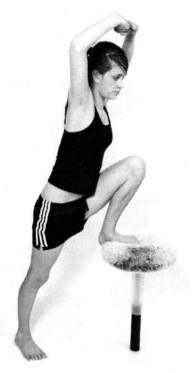

1. <u>Bend your elbows</u> and bring your hands together above your head. (Don't give up. This is a little challenging to do while moving your body forward)
2. <u>Bend left knee</u> and keep your left foot on the secured support.
3. Keeping your back straight move your upper body forward towards your left knee. (Feel it in the lower, mid and upper back)
4. Inhale deeply and exhale while stretching your spine upwards.
5. Hold position 5 seconds. Do once.

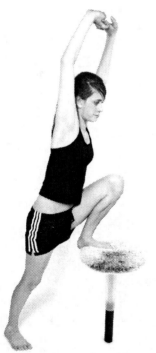

6. Keep prior position with your upper body forward and left knee bent.
7. <u>Stretch your arms up holding your hands together.</u> (Feel it in the lower, mid and upper back)
8. Inhale deeply and exhale while stretching your spine upwards.
9. Hold position 5 seconds. Do once.

Repeat *Legs Up Phase I and II* with the right leg.

Chest Out (In front of mirror)

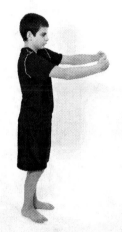 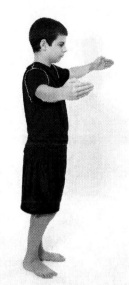 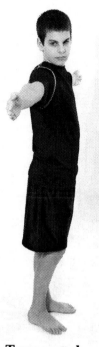

1. **Bring your arms forward at shoulder length and join your hands in front of you.**

2. **Keep your chest out as you bring your arms out slowly.**

3. **Turn your head to the right side as you open your arms.** (Feel it between your shoulder blades)

4. **Repeat while turning your head to the other side.**

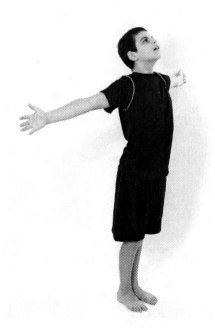

5. **Finish *Chest Out* by bringing head to the center and slightly back.**
   (Feel it between the shoulder blades, as you stretch your arms gently back as far as you can reach)

6. **Inhale. Exhale.**

7. **Bring your arms to the sides.**

8. **Relax.**

The reason I like to call this next movement ***Bonsai Tree*** is to serve as a reminder that if the tree (the spine) is curved to the wrong side, you need to bend it the opposite way. In this case the model is bending to the right side, against *his* curve. (Check page 21 if you are not sure)

Bonsai Tree

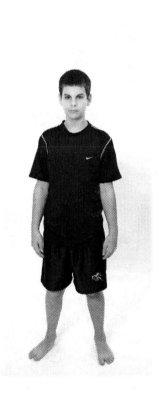 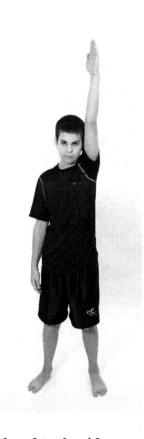 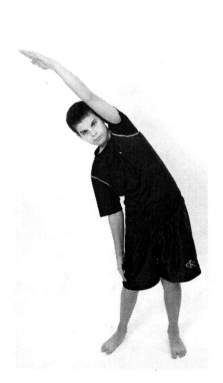

1. **Face the mirror with hands relaxed to the sides.**
2. **Use the mirror to see that shoulders are straight.**
3. **Place feet apart slightly more than shoulders width.**
4. **Keep knees relaxed.**
5. **Inhale as you bring one arm straight up to your ear. Stretch as high as you can.**
6. **Keep the other hand at your side.**
   (Feel the stretch of the muscles from your feet to your fingers as you bend your spine against the curve, the high end)
7. **Exhale as you bend as far as you can. Keep elbow straight and breathe regularly.**
8. **Do not twist body.**
9. **Do not bend elbow.**
10. **Breathe regularly as you hold position for 5 seconds.**
11. **Return to center and repeat 3 times to "your" side.**

Bonsai Sway

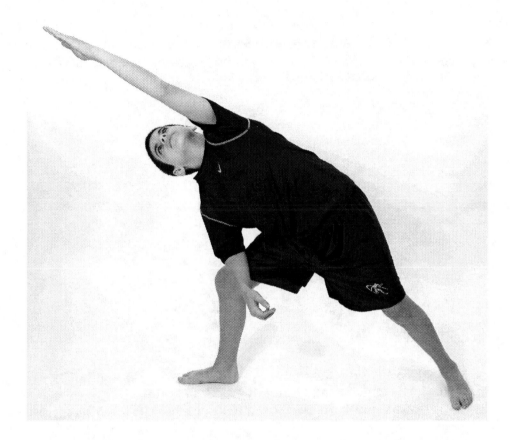

1. **From the last upright position, bring your left leg straight out to the side.**
2. **Bend your right knee and place your foot facing forward as you bend in the same direction.**
3. **Bring your left arm straight up above head.**
4. **You can use the right arm on your upper right leg if you need some support.**
5. **Look up. Hold position 5 seconds.** (Feel your spine bending against the curve, the high end)
6. **Maintain your balance and keeping your right arm above your head, while you switch legs by bending your left knee and stretching your right leg out by your side.**
7. **Sway on your legs 5 times** (from one side to the other) **without bringing your arm down or changing the direction of your back being bent to "your" side.**

"Everyday I learn something new. I like that."

Jessie (15 years old) 2007

Using Weights

Use the appropriate weights for your present fitness; 3 to 5 pounds is usually the norm for someone just starting out. Try to maintain your back flat against the floor. (Feel the gentle stretch between your shoulders with each time you bring your elbows down to start again)

One

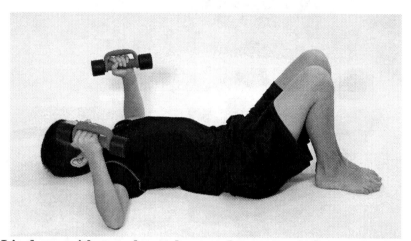

1. Lie down with your knees bent and your back flat on the floor.
2. Hold the weights facing each other as in the photo.
3. Your elbows should be paralleled to your shoulders at 90 degrees.

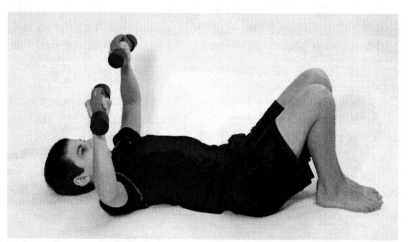

4. Keeping elbows slightly bent, bring weights up while rotating your wrists 90 degrees.
5. The back of your hands should be facing you, as in the photo.
6. Each time the weights join above your head, count one rep.
   (Feel the gentle stretch between your shoulders each time you bring your elbows down to start again) **Repeat 10 times, slowly.**

Two

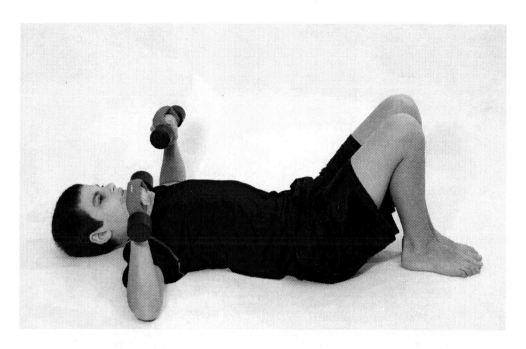

1. Have your elbows bent and paralleled to your shoulders at 90 degrees.

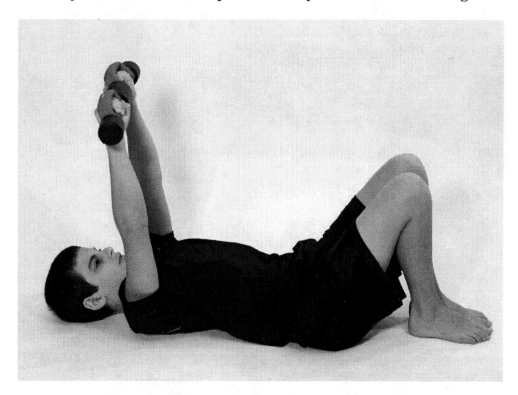

2. Raise the weights straight up in line with your shoulders.
3. Keep your back flat on the floor.
4. Repeat 10 times.

Three

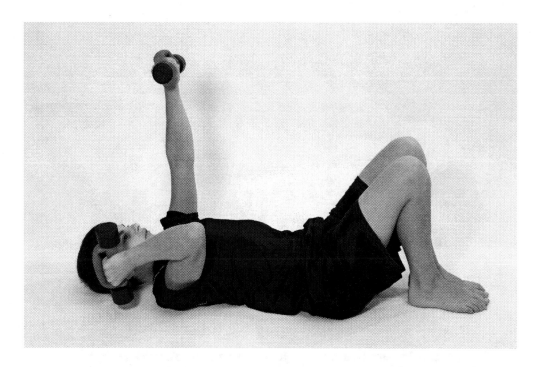

1. Beginning from the last position, bend one arm at the elbow and bring the weight to the side of your head.
2. Keep your back flat against the floor.

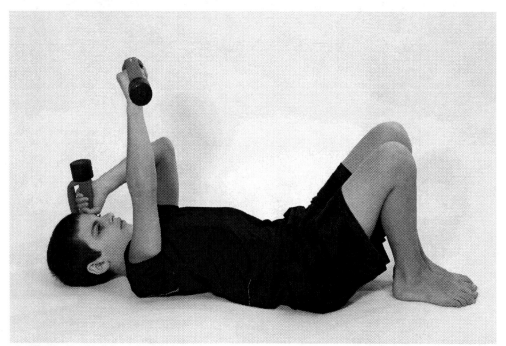

3. Switch to the other arm.
4. Repeat 10 times to each side.

Side to Side – Rotation

As you rotate your spine slowly from one side to the other use the weight (can be a small ball, or anything that is easy to lift) **close to your body. This movement keeps your spine flexible by retaining side-to-side mobility and tones the surrounding muscles. Feel it around your waist.**

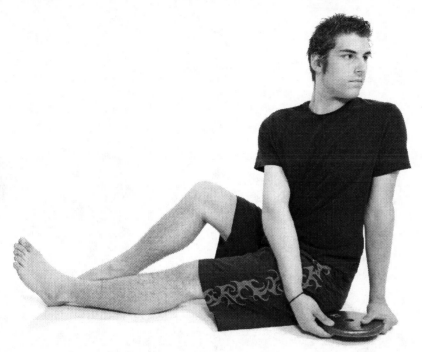

Can be done seated on the floor. I prefer to use a chair. (Keep weight close to your body)

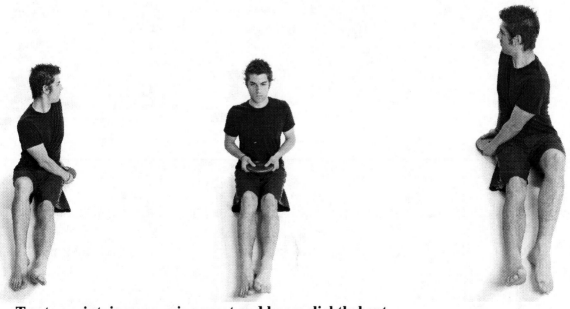

1. **Try to maintain your spine erect and knees slightly bent.**
2. **Repeat 10 times to each side.**

Give me Five

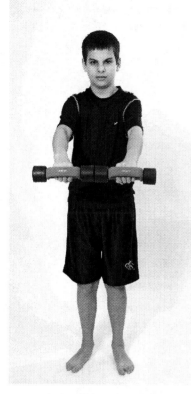

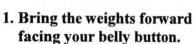

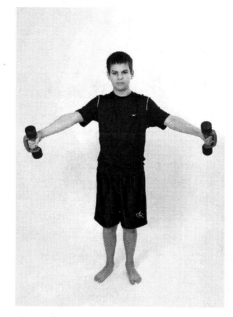

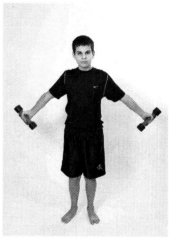

1. **Bring the weights forward facing your belly button.**

2. **Maintain the same distance all around as you bring your arms out to the sides.**

3. **Bring your arms back gently as you pull your chest out.**
4. **Hold 5 seconds.** (Feel it across your mid and upper back)
5. **Repeat 5 times.**

"Inside of a ring or out, ain't nothing wrong with going down. It's staying down that's wrong."

Muhammad Ali

Use Your Own Weight

If you do not have access to a local gym, you may want to inquire about a pull up bar that can be securely installed in one of the doorways in your home.

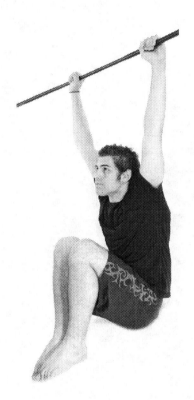

1. Grasp the bar with both hands and allow your entire body weight to hang down.
2. Hold for 5 seconds while relaxing your back.
3. Try not to swing.
4. Bring knees up as high as you can.
5. Concentrate. Let your abdominal muscles help you out.
6. Try a minimum of 3 times or until you are unable to bring knees up.

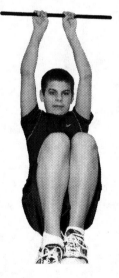

I highly recommend swimming, using free style and or breaststroke, **at least twice a week.**
At the end of swimming for half-an-hour try using the deep end of the pool to allow your spine to stretch down as you hold on to the edge of the pool. Hold for 10 seconds and then curl up by bringing your knees to your chest as if you are hanging from a pull up bar and hold for another10 seconds. Do that as many times as you like.

Desk Stretch One

Are you overdoing it at the computer? Spending too much time in a seated position? After an hour seated, try the following for a quick stretch of the spine.

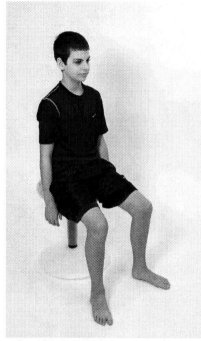

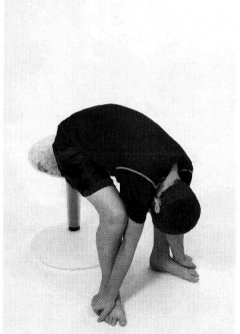

1. Sit straight with your hands relaxed at sides.
2. Take a deep breath, exhale and relax.

3. Let your body drop slowly forward until you reach your ankles.
(Feel the stretch throughout your spine from the lower back to your neck and shoulders)

4. Return slowly to the upright position.
5. Take a deep breath as you come up.
6. Repeat twice.

Desk Stretch Two

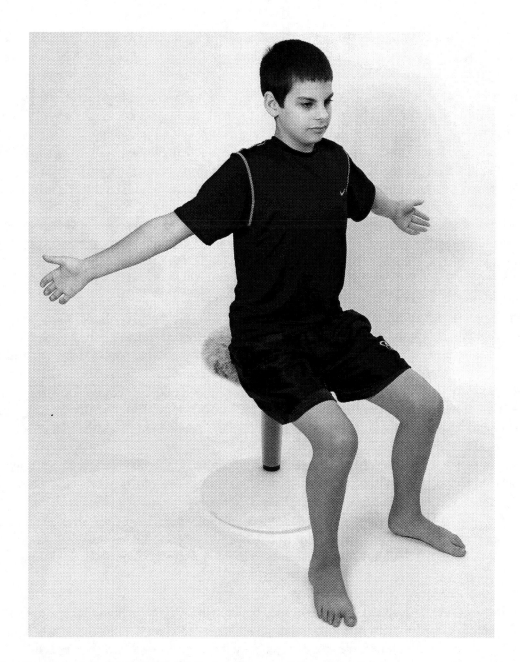

1. **Reach behind you with both arms away from your body.**
2. **Rotate palms up. Hold for 5 seconds.**
   (Feel your chest and the front of your shoulders stretching as you tighten
   the mid and upper back)
3. **Relax your arms to the sides and down.**
4. **Take a deep breath. Exhale.**
5. **Repeat 3 times.**

Affirmations and Goals

An affirmation is a positive thought. We need positive thoughts every day of our lives because once we start to have negative ideas, it is no different then giving up.

While driving to work, I have gotten used to giving thanks for everything I have, including my luck to live in these modern times and have a car to get to work and not a covered wagon. Other times, I give thanks for having eyeglasses to see and one ear still working. Everything counts. In the winter, I am grateful for the heat in the car and in the summer time I feel blessed with an air conditioner that works. At the end of a day's work I give thanks for the privilege of working side by side with my son and having done my best to help people to recover their health. At the end of a day's work, I can't wait to go home and see my husband. I give thanks for having arms to hug him back.

In the morning I make affirmations like, "Today is going to be awesome." And I smile at everyone I meet, because I know it is contagious. I like being surrounded by happy, healthy people. I can't help myself, it feels good to see someone leaving our office feeling better and looking forward to a more productive life.

An affirmation can be about anything that we want to turn out positive, like, "I am great at math. I love math and anything with numbers is going to be absorbed into my brain like a sponge of knowledge by the end of the day, as I will work hard at making it happen." Okay, so this is a huge affirmation, but the bigger the better, it gives more room to play.

Here are some more examples, use your own words "I will do something kind for a friend," or "Today I will eat some fresh vegetables at dinner," or "As of today, I will not drink any more soda." An affirmation can be a goal towards personal growth like, "As of today I am patient," or "I am going to start eating healthy."

Go ahead, stick a note on the refrigerator, or your closet door, and make it visual, so you can read it every day until you succeed. Without action, it's only words. The old proverb *God helps those that help themselves* has proven to be true to many successful people.

Nobody is going to knock at your door and hand you an education or a job. You need to go out there and get it yourself. If you are successful in reaching your goal, treat yourself to a gift at the end of the month, or donate some money to help someone in need. Give random gifts of kindness.

Giving thanks for everything we have develops naturally with each day we grow, even if we have to loose something in order to appreciate it. It is sad, but it is true. Remember, success doesn't come to us. It comes *from* us. Our thoughts create the reality we live in and our actions make it happen. Turning fear into confidence and lessons to be learned is not easy but if you say, *I can* then *you will*.

Place this book in the room where you will most likely be doing **TESP** on a daily basis and take the first step towards helping yourself.

"THINK! SPEAK! ACT POSITIVE! I AM! I WILL! I CAN! I MUST!"

B.J. Palmer, D.C.

Food for Wellness

(Healthy diet = Healthier spine)

Why is our diet so important? Because we are what we eat! Many of us think of this statement as just an old proverb, but the truth is that what goes into our system becomes part of it. The proper diet is vital in providing the nutrients needed to make us grow and maintain our health.

A study from researchers in Washington D.C. found that "nutrition should logically be considered as a possible factor in human Scoliosis, based in part by a review of all of the animal studies where nutrition plays a role in the disorder." Studies were performed on animals by exposing them to toxins like drugs, pesticides and foods deficient in certain vitamins. [1] The study concluded "there is evidence that poor nutrition may play a role in the etiology (*the cause*) of Idiopathic Scoliosis. This possibility should be examined further in humans."

A few years ago, I was visiting a friend who is a working mom. She was serving the kids their dinner when I stopped over. They were having hot dogs. That was their dinner. She told me that chicken fingers were their favorite, but she didn't have time to pick those up on the way home. I didn't know that chickens have fingers. I took my little niece to day-care a few times and one morning I got there as they were about to serve breakfast, waffles covered with canned fruit in sugary syrup. Is it really a surprise that the USA, one of the most powerful countries in the world, is rated 35th when it comes to health care? There are 35 other countries where the citizens are healthier than we are!

Healthy habits have to start at a young age if we are going to build a future of Wellness. If bones loose their health they may become brittle or soft, and as we age the spine will continue to deteriorate. We already have enough to deal with from our DNA; breaking the family mold of diabetes, heart disease, and so many other health issues that are now running rampant through the USA. Let's make a change. It's a question of good habits starting out early in life.

Because what we eat does influence our bones and of course our health, I have enclosed some information on osteoporosis. It may sound like a long time from now for anyone that is in their teens to start worrying about their aging bones. But osteoporosis is no longer associated only with old age; Scoliosis in some cases can be affected by osteoporosis at a young age. I hope that as you read on, you will understand that healthy habits can make a difference for when you grow up.

[1]Nutri-Kinetics in Washington, D.C. published in J Manipulative Physiology. Therapy 1993 Mar-Apr; 16 (3): 69 – 73 "Nutrition as a environmental factor in the etiology of Idiopathic Scoliosis." Worthington V. Shambaugh P.

Fast Food versus a Home Made Meal

These are some of the excuses people use for eating fast food and hardly ever making an effort to make a home cooked meal: "I don't want to cook just for myself, it's not worth all that work," "I am too tired to cook," "I don't know how to cook, I can't even boil water," "I know fast food is not good but…we have to die from something, don't we?"

Yes, but why do we have to clog our arteries on the way out? What's wrong with inviting ourselves to a daily private celebration? Yes, daily invitation! Aren't we worth it?

If you are into science or into analytical things, think of preparing food as a wonderful and exciting technical experiment. Give it some thought, like "Let's see what I can produce out of mixing half a cup of that and adding an ounce of this and a teaspoon of that" or … if you are an artist, "Let's see what sensational creation I can put together out of mixing these colors with those darker greens and a touch of those herbs and just a dab of mixed nuts." You don't have to use those exact words.☺

Because of the pressure society puts on all of us, when it comes to having everything we want for our family or simply making ends meet, most adults have to work fulltime and sometimes our young people get home and there's nobody there. It comes down to staring at the refrigerator hoping something will materialize into a meal. Finally one gives up and opts for a quick bowl of sugary, dry cereal or a pop tart from the toaster. This can happen to us even when we are on our own or in college and we figure "so what, four or six years of junk food is not going to kill me."

Guess what, it does have an impact on our health even if it takes a couple of years before we notice the changes. Ask a college student upon graduation what has happened to them along the way.

Who said going to school is not work and what about the stress most students experience? If they didn't take care of themselves they got fat, their hair may have thinned, they look older; their health is not what used to be. If you are still in denial concerning fast food, rent the movie "Super Size Me" and see what happened to somebody else.

I believe the beginning of our lives can produce the end result of our health and who we will become. The old motto *we are what we eat* has become a concrete reality for me through seeing young patients who are not only obese, but also carry a multitude of health problems that have "developed" during their growing years.

One particular case comes to mind. A 14-year-old boy came into our office to have a sports physical. He was about 50 lbs overweight. When he took his shirt off, he sat consciously aware of his looks, while folding his arms across his chest. At the end of the physical exam I encouraged him to talk about his present situation. I found out that his mom and sister had the same weight problem, but when it came to shopping for food he was at the mercy of whatever was available at home.

I spoke to his mom and we all agreed that it wasn't going to be easy. She was encouraged to see a Naturopathic Physician who could guide their family in a proper diet.

Healthy Hints

1. Get a diabetic cookbook for some ideas on healthy eating and portions. Borrow one from the library if you don't have the budget.
2. Buy organic food. If you can't afford organic food, inquire if what you are buying has been sprayed with insecticides, herbicides, or fungicides.
3. If you can't pronounce an ingredient, it's not food.
4. My favorite cooking books are from Hernes House Publications and they are sold at Borders. I enjoy their full-page pictures of mouth-watering recipes with a list of ingredients needed and step-by-step color picture instruction.
5. When ordering a pizza, ask for light cheese and veggies instead of greasy sausages and meat.
6. Combo meals sound like a wallet savings but the calories go right around your waist.
7. Giving up on fast food is not easy for many people, but you can still make the right choices by ordering the salad with the light dressing on the side. You control how much dressing you really need.
8. Make sure they add the lettuce and tomato to your sandwich or burger and ask them to skip on the special sauce, mayonnaise, cheese and bacon.
9. Choose grilled versus fried. Less oil = less fat and calories.
10. A kid's meal goes a long way, try it next time, you will be surprised how big it is.
11. I believe most people already know this factoid but here it goes. If you eat before shopping for food, you will be less likely to buy on impulse because it "looks" good.
12. It's also a great idea to make a list of what you need, and buy ONLY what is ON THAT LIST!
13. Read the ingredients on food labels. Pick the foods with shorter lists; the longer the list, the more likely that what you are buying is full of additives, preservatives, and artificial colors.

Once in a while, go with your mom or dad shopping for food and offer some suggestions for healthy snacks. Most parents are pleased to know that their kids don't want just junk food.

Get involved in the kitchen. Someday when you are on your own, you will be able to take care of yourself. Think of it as an apprenticeship towards your own future, not to mention that your family will appreciate your help.

**Life can often be compared
to a stained glass window.
You can choose your panes,
and make it more beautiful.**

Danlar

Snacks for all ages

Here are some ideas from young people for munchies to take to school, as well as a couple of easy recipes for when you get home and sometimes you have to wait until dinner is ready.

Jacob, 13: Says he loves the taste of green apples, and fresh broccoli and carrots. He shared his secret on how he makes his favorite snack. He leaves the fresh corn in its husk, wraps it in a moist paper towel and microwaves it for 4 minutes.

Shayna, 11: Likes easy to prepare snacks like: baby carrots, celery, watermelon, peaches, and plums.

Connor, 15: Loves potatoes, especially the red ones; he uses the microwave when he gets home to cook a medium sized one, then he adds some salt and lemon pepper to taste. His other favorite snacks are soft pretzels topped with mustard and air-popped popcorn.

Ben, 17: Is a vegetarian. He loves raw vegetables. His favorite salad is a mix of fresh spinach and other greens with olive oil, balsamic vinegar, crushed fresh garlic, salt, and pepper to taste. Sometimes he adds walnuts and sliced oranges on top of the salad.

Mark, 14: His favorite is pita bread stuffed with cut-up banana, almond butter, and sliced apples, his grandmother used to make it for him when he was younger. He also enjoys granola with yogurt.

Roselyn and her sister Stacy, 14 & 15: Their favorite food is a burrito sandwich of rolled up turkey, lettuce and tomato in a flour tortilla. During avocado season, they like to add a few slices to the burrito ingredients. This is their own personal recipe for a summer drink: in a blender, combine ½ cup each of your favorite fruit juice, (it has to be 100% fruit juice, they said), plain yogurt, and fresh fruit. (They both love berries and banana) Add a few ice cubes. Blend until smooth.

Molly, 13: Enjoys fresh sliced apples dipped in peanut butter. She also likes steamed broccoli and real cheddar cheese. She says this is a special treat and she doesn't over do it with the cheddar cheese

Amy, 16: Makes her own trail mix of pine nuts, almonds, raisins, dried apricots, and cranberries to take to school.

Whenever possible, eat foods that are alive with colors. The colors indicate that you are getting lots of different minerals and vitamins.

Surviving College (Living on your own)

If your refrigerator has *nothing* inside, you are far more likely to open a can of something or go out for fast food, meaning its quality and contents are questionable. Some suggestions for those days when opening the refrigerator and you wish there was *something* ready to eat.

Boiled eggs (boil a half a dozen or more once a month, they keep for weeks in the refrigerator).
Non-fat cottage cheese.
Turkey bacon.
Broiled fish or chicken (If cooked with a little soy sauce, the leftovers are great cold and they make great sandwiches).
Soups (without cream).
Low fat cheese, such as mozzarella string cheese.
Vegetables, and hummus or low-fat dressing for dipping. (I personally like my veggies plain)
Apple sauce or other fruit cups (packed in fruit juice, not syrup).
Various containers in the freezer with homemade meals ready to eat.

Oh, those days of college, what a learning experience! Is it any different from when you are in high school or on a job from nine to five? No, it all comes down to one question; "What's there to eat?"

What one learns in school goes beyond the classroom, as you tend to survive in a world of personal choices! Sunday morning was my shopping day for general groceries. I carried a list of items that covered every meal needed for the week. Each recipe was made with one goal in mind, how many meals could I make out of a single large one? How many meals could I make out of the vegetable stew, the lasagna, or the large pot of green soup? The containers were filled and frozen, and sometimes the Sundays went by and I had no need to shop or cook for several weeks because I had enough frozen containers to feed an army. I always had a small bowl of fresh green salad with dinner.

If you don't have someone to cook for you, guess what; it's time to learn. If you were in a shipwreck and found yourself in a deserted island, would you sit cross-legged by the ocean and wait until someone came by with hamburgers or would you immediately assess the situation and get to work? Yeah, you'd better start building some form of shelter and don't forget those coconuts above your head, use them to their full potential. Besides making excellent fresh coconut pies, you can also use them to knock a rabbit out and make yourself a barbeque under the moonlight or just keep him as your buddy.

If you are younger than 18 years old do not attempt this unless you have parental supervision. If you are 18 or older, get yourself a wok. If you can't afford a new one, get it used for a few dollars at a thrift store. It's the quickest and easiest way to stir fry a quick meal for yourself or the entire family. Always use extra virgin olive oil to coat the pan first and then add fresh vegetables, fresh herbs, and garlic or onion, tofu, or small pieces of chicken without skin.

Stone Soup

Someone may want to ask what does *stone soup* have to do with the management of Scoliosis. The answer is quite simple. It is a true story according to my Aunt Heydee, who used to entertain my brothers and me with stories from a long, long time ago. She said if it was not for *stone soup* there would be no *green soup* today. Since children need to eat their vegetables in order to get the proper nutrition for their bones, the *stone soup* story is an important historical event. Second, it teaches us to never give up, because no matter how bad the odds are, while there is life there is hope.

The will power to stay focused in your goals is what is going to make a difference, if you can control Scoliosis or is it going to control you. Nothing is impossible unless you give up.

Once upon a time, a beggar was walking through Siberia. Now, everybody knows that Siberia is in Russia and it is very cold there. After days and days of walking in the snow, the beggar reached a little town where he hoped to find some food. He was not only cold, but he was also very hungry. He knocked on somebody's door and asked for a piece of bread and a bowl of hot soup.

The answer was, "Sorry fellow, we only have a couple of onions and nothing else to eat. Leave us alone."

And so he crossed the street to the next house and they closed the door on him after saying, "Sorry fellow, we only have a couple of potatoes for our dinner tonight. Now scram."

He went from door to door and it was always the same answer, they didn't have enough food to share with him. Not ready to give up, he sat down by the only well in the center of the small town and for a while just sat there shaking as he felt himself freezing under the cold winter wind of Siberia. Then he had an idea, he brought the water pail up from the well, half full. With his last match he still had in his coat pocket, he began a little fire with the help of a couple of sticks. He settled the pail of water on the burning wood and watched as it started to boil. The people in the village could see him through their windows and wondered what he was doing. They came out of their houses to see up close.

He threw a couple of stones into the water pail and said, "You are all welcome to have some of my stone soup with me, because I have plenty to share with you, but you know what," he said, turning to one of the village women watching him, "If you were as kind as to bring me a couple of potatoes to add to the stone soup, I bet you would enjoy this soup a lot more."

One of the villagers watching said, "I am hungry, and so is my wife. Do you mind if I bring some dandelions and a couple of onions and you share your delicious stone soup with us?"

Little by little, everyone was bringing something to add to the stone soup, which came to be what we know today as *green soup,* (the recipe follows in the next page without the stones of course) the most nourishing and awesome soup the villagers in that forsaken place had ever had. From that day on, *stone soup* became a regular part of their daily diet and everybody lived happily ever after, because they learned to share their food with each other and nobody went hungry ever again.

Strength comes from adversity, power comes from changing lives for the better.

Danlar

Green Soup

Due to popular demand, here is the famous *"green soup"* recipe. Children and adults love to eat it, even if they don't like vegetables. My two sons used to love this soup when they were children, and they still do.

In a pot (a large pot is a good idea if you are going to make extra soup for another day) cover with water 10 carrots, 2 turnips (if your market has more than one kind, get one of each) 2 large onions, 3 potatoes, a bunch of spinach, a good stalk of broccoli, 3 stalks of celery, a handful of parsley, fresh garlic, some chard leafs, a beef bone and salt to taste. (If you are a vegetarian add a few cubes of concentrated veggie broth instead of the bone.)
Let it cook until all the contents are soft. Use a masher to turn the soup into a loose puree and all clues of vegetable preexistence are basically out of sight.

Without using the bone, this recipe is especially good for someone trying to lose weight. Babies love the texture. Children can't resist it if you add the alphabet pasta to the creamy soup. Anyone looking to increase their calcium intake is encouraged to chop collard greens very thin and add them to the creamy soup to cook until tender.

For a variety in taste, add chickpeas, red beans, cabbage, elbow macaroni, the combinations can be endless, just like *stone soup*.

HINT: If when you finish eating you feel energized, you have eaten the appropriate nutrients for your body, if you feel tired and sluggish after a meal, then you had the wrong food or overburdened the body with too much.

Eat to live - Don't live to eat.

– Anonymous

Organic Food

Farmer markets are becoming ever more popular with the general public and supermarkets are now starting to offer organic fruits, vegetables and meats. Yes, the price is sometimes higher than the chemical sprayed items we have been buying all these years, but educated consumers have been putting enough pressure on the food industry and the prices are slowly but surely becoming more affordable.

Organic foods taste great because farmers do not use genetically engineered seeds or crops, chemical fertilizer, sewage sludge, pesticides, herbicides or fungicides in growing it. Livestock is treated humanely and are not given antibiotics or artificial growth hormones. They are provided organically grown feed, fresh air, and outdoor access. Food processing does not contain genetically modified ingredients or synthetic preservatives.

Want to know more?
Visit www.organic-center.org

The Organic Center is a friendly site with the latest news about food quality and an extensive consumer guide. Their mission is "To generate credible, peer reviewed scientific information and communicate the verifiable benefits of organic farming and products to society."
   Stay informed with their monthly e-newsletter, *The Scoop*!

For a comprehensive look at the USDA Organic Rules, organic agriculture, the organic industry and why they are committed to providing organic products in their store check out www.wholefoodsmarket.com

For specific information about the Organic Rule, contact the USDA's National Organic Program at 202-720-3252 or visit www.ams.usda.gov/nop.

The US Centers for Disease Control estimate that the average family spends 40 percent of its food budget on fast food.

"You must be the change you wish to see in the world."

Mohandas Gandhi

Fruits and Vegetables

Unless you have your own fruit trees growing in your back yard, fruit should be bought to last no more than three days since you want them to be rich in flavor and freshness. Always wash fruit before eating it, and have it handy to take with you to school, work, or as a snack when you get home and need something to hold you until dinner is ready.

If you have a backyard big enough to plant a fruit tree, consider planting a mini tree, it's easier than most people think, and relatively inexpensive. A fig tree doesn't like water; imagine no watering, no garden work. Grapes grow along a sunny fence as well as blueberries and strawberries, and none of these like to be fussed with. Outside my office, I have a dwarf tree that grows Asian pears and apples. I call it my garden dessert.

Check out some garden farms and see what they have to offer. Most of the time they are eager to help you to get creative with whatever garden space you have available. If you live in the city, your neighbors may be more than glad to start a community garden.

My roommate Sara and I lived in an apartment complex where there was no room to plant anything except some herbs on the kitchen sill. One day, she went to a thrift shop and bought three large, tall laundry baskets. She lined the baskets with heavy-duty plastic garbage bags and filled them with dirt, and then she planted a few tomato plants.

We had so many tomatoes growing that summer that we shared them with friends at college.

If you like fruit juice or vegetable juice try to drink it in moderation. While in Chiropractic College I started juicing every morning, especially carrots. One day one of our professors mentioned in class that juicing was not as beneficial as many people thought because we were only drinking the juice and missing out on the natural fiber that whole vegetables and fruits provide. He added that we were also increasing our calories and overburdening our system. He gave us the example of eating a normal portion of one or two whole carrots versus drinking eight to ten carrots for a glass of juice with little fiber.

Of course I was not going to stop drinking my morning carrot juice and if anything I increased the dosage by drinking another glass of tasty sweet refreshing carrot juice as soon as I got home.

Not too long afterwards I was in lab with other students practicing physical exams on each other and one student looked at the palm of my hands and commented, "Wow! Your hands are orange! Matter of a fact, even your face is orange, what's wrong with your skin?"

The carotene from the carrots was coming out through my skin!

Start by doing what's necessary, then what's possible,
and suddenly you are doing the impossible.

– Saint Francis of Assisi

Low Fat Plain Yogurt

Get plain yogurt without sugary jam fruit or additives. You control what you add to it, with goodies like honey, or fruit in season like berries, mangoes, bananas, chopped nuts, grapes, and so on.

An *almost* guiltless dessert:

You will need strawberries or any other in season berry which you like, and low-fat plain yogurt. Wash the strawberries, take their stems off, and slice them. Sprinkle them with a very small amount of brown sugar. Put them in a tight container and refrigerate them over night. Take a look the next day, and notice that you now have rich strawberry juice and strawberries that have transformed into sweet tasty morsels with an aroma to kill for.
Fill a cup of yogurt and mix two good spoonfuls of the juice and strawberries into it.

* When mangos are in season, they hardly ever need any sugar. They are also a great fruit to add to plain yogurt. Apples and bananas shouldn't be prepared a day before, they are better if eaten upon being freshly cut.

Another guiltless dessert:

In a small, deep bowl, put about three quarters of a cup of frozen berries (Costco sells a mix of raspberries, blueberries and marionberries) microwave it for one minute. Take out the bowl and sprinkle with two or three tablespoons of granola and microwave for one more minute. Add to the bowl a small cup of low-fat plain yogurt. Add a dash of cinnamon if you like.

Soy, Rice or Almond Milk

(Most people with lactose intolerance know this already.)

Bread (Read the ingredients if you are allergic to wheat or gluten.)

My favorite bread is Dave's Killer Bread, easily found in the health isle at most grocery stores. It keeps well in the freezer and it's already sliced and ready for the toaster. I like it plain.
It's also great with cheese, jam and/or peanut or almond butter with a hint of honey, a real tasty treat. A glass of juice or milk along with it is perfect. Visit www.Daveskillerbread.com to find out more.

Vegetarianism

The health benefits associated with eating more vegetables and fruit and less meat have been proven with studies that show clearly a decreased risk for diabetes, some types of cancer, obesity and heart diseases. Still, I must mention that all young-people considering a vegetarian life style should be under observation with a Naturopath or a nutritionist to make sure they are following a proper diet. Through the years, I have encountered a few teen patients that became vegetarians at a very young age. These young patients showed depleted signs of important minerals in their body and were also at a high risk for hormonal deficiencies and developmental issues. Because of this I am putting extra emphasis on good nutrition and encouraging you to do further research on this topic before making such an important decision concerning your health. Moderation is the key to everything; beef fat won't kill you if it is an occasional indulgence.

If you are contemplating becoming a vegetarian the following are necessary to maintain optimum health:

Calcium - broccoli, kale, collard, yogurt, okra, dairy, tofu, soymilk, almonds, dried figs, legumes.

Protein - beans, lentils, tempeh, tofu and other soy-based meat substitutes, dairy, eggs.

Vitamin D - sunshine, vitamin D supplements, fortified cow's milk, soymilk and cereals.

Iron - chickpeas, lentils, adzuki and kidney beans, cashews, almonds, dark leafy greens such as spinash.

Zinc - adzuki and navy beans, split peas, cashews, pumpkin and sunflower seeds, soy foods.

Vitamin B12 - from B12 supplements, nutritional yeast- delicious on popcorn, fortified cereals with Vitamin B12 like Enriched Bran Flakes. I don't mean Captain Crunch ☺

Iodide - from iodized salt, kelp powder and other sea vegetables.

Essential Fatty Acids - from direct sources such as microalgae supplements, Albacore tuna, seaweed and salmon, which have high levels of omega-3 fatty acids. Secondary sources include flaxseed oil, hempseed oil, walnuts and canola oil.

- Check out the *List of Foods High in Essential Nutrients* on page 79.

Foods to avoid or decrease consumption:

Fried foods, caffeine, large amounts of bread and pasta, most products ending in -etos, or -itos like Cheetos, Fritos, Doritos, and so on. Read the labels. Ingredients that sound more like chemistry experiment, foods with trans fats, or where the word "hydrogenated" appears on the package should be avoid.

Products that are sweet or salty are likely over sweetened or over salted. This is because salt and sugar is used to help improve taste, just like oil is over used to make food taste better at poor quality restaurants.

Good Hygiene Habits are Very Important

A few years ago I learned how easy it is to get food poisoning if not careful. I was mixing some ground meat into meatballs and decided to add some fresh spinach to it. I used my hands several times to grab the spinach from a bowl as I added it to the ground meat. After I was done mixing the meatballs I put away the fresh spinach, which I served in a salad the next day for dinner. Not a good idea! Food poisoning was the result of touching the spinach without washing my hands after handling raw meat.

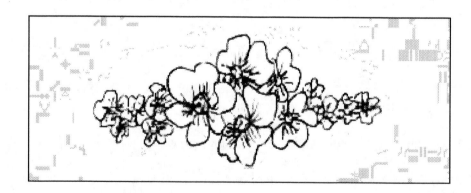

List of Foods High In Essential Nutrients

Vitamin A
(For the eyes and skin)

Liver
Dark green leafy veggies
Apricots
Nectarines
Cantaloupe
Sweet potatoes
Eggs
Squash
Carrots
Spinach, Chard
Tomato

Thiamin (Vitamin B1)
(Improves mental function)

Yeast, brewer's
Yeast, torula
Wheat germ
Sunflower seeds
Rice polishings
Pine nuts
Beans, pinto & red
Peanuts, with skins
Brazil nuts
Pecans
Soybean flour

Vitamin C
(For strong teeth, gums, and bones)

Brussel sprouts
Guava
Broccoli
Green pepper
Cantaloupe
Dark green leafy
Brussels sprouts
Citrus fruit or juice
Fresh strawberries
Cabbage
Watermelon

Zinc
(Immune and sensory)

Oysters, fresh
Pumpkin seeds
Oats
Ginger root
Pecans
Split peas, dry
Brazil nuts
Peanuts
Rye
Whole-wheat

Vitamin K
(Helps with blood clotting)

Dark green leafy veggies
Broccoli
Baked beans
Spinach
Lettuce
Cabbage
Cheese
Soybeans
Safflower oil
Egg yokes

Vitamin E
(Protects the tissues and oxygen utilization)

Soybean oil
Corn
Cottonseed oil
Wheat germ
Peanuts
Mayonnaise
Broiled salmon
Asparagus
Cauliflower
Dark leafy

Iron
(For healthy blood)

Eggs
Baked beans
Liver
Prune juice
Apricots
Raisins
Spinach
Soybeans

Selenium
(Antioxidant function)

Garlic, Brown rice
Orange juice
Wheat germ
Brazil nuts
Oats, Bran
Whole-wheat bread
Barley, Turnips
Tuna, herring

Potassium
(For muscle, nerves and energy)

Baked beans
Halibut, Beef
Soybeans
Cantaloupe
Sweet potatoes
Avocado, Molasses
Raisins, Ham
Banana, Mushrooms

Water

(The best thirst quencher - ever)

If you have doubts about what water can do for a living organism, get yourself a small house plant and put it inside a gorgeous ceramic container in your favorite room. Watch what happens to that plant when you forget to water it for a few days.

If lack of water (dehydration) caused the plant to dry and shrivel up guess what happens to us when we don't drink enough water. The experts say that dehydration is the leading cause of premature aging. I believe it!

75% of Americans are chronically dehydrated.
(Likely applies to half the world population)

A mere 2% drop in body water can cause fuzzy short-term memory, trouble with basic math, and difficulty focusing on the computer screen or a printed page.

Lack of water is the #1 trigger of daytime fatigue.

73% of your body is water.

Drinking 5 glasses of water daily decreases the risk of colon cancer by 45% and also makes one less likely to develop bladder cancer.

Water makes up more than half your body composition and must be replenished daily! Your skin loses water every day through perspiration. The lungs need about two glasses of water each day in order to function properly. The small intestines need water to promote elimination and the kidneys also need a large quantity of water daily to carry out wastes. The discs in our spine, which are located between each vertebra as a soft cushion, are 85% made of water. We need those discs!

After the age of 35 years old we start to loose the ability to sense that we are dehydrated.

Some ideas for putting a bit of flavor in your water: Freeze some freshly squeezed lemon juice, grapefruit or orange juice into an ice cube tray and drop it into your tall glass of water. Drink it along with your meal, instead of soda pop, or juice.

• Are you wondering if your drink enough water daily? Here is a marker, if you don't urinate at least every four hours when you are awake; you need to increase your water intake. Most likely you are dehydrated.

Distilled vs Bottled vs Tap vs Filtered Water

Distilled water ……………………………………Lack of naturally-occurring minerals.

Bottled water……………………………………The Food and Drug Administration (FDA) does not define guidelines for which regulations may be considered applicable, nor set requirements for water sources in the absence of applicable laws. Additionally, bottled water suppliers are not required to provide details of the water source on the labels. Water bottlers are not required to test for E. Coli, cryptosporidium, giardia, asbestos, or certain organic compounds such as benzenes.

Tap water………………………………………..Plastic piping has been in wide use for the domestic water supply since the 1970s. The main problems associated with tap water are: chlorine, fluoride, cancer-causing agents like PCBs, THMs, heavy metals. Nobody knows how many toxic chemicals may actually be in tap water.

A recent Ralph Nader Report stated, "After reviewing over 10,000 pages of Environmental Protection Agency (EPA) documents acquired through the Freedom Of information Act, over 2300 chemicals that cause cancer have been detected in U.S. tap water."

Filtered water……………………………………Is less expensive than bottled water and you are in charge of its quality and purity by picking the filter system that suits your needs.

Try to use glass to store filtered water. If glass is not practical to store water and you have to use plastic; translucent, colored, or bottles with a number other than 1 on the bottom should be avoided because of the risk of chemicals leeching into the water from the plastic.

Drink water for good health. It's wholesome.
No calories, no fat.

Soft Drinks

A 1994 issue of the "Journal of Adolescent Health" study concluded, "The high consumption of carbonated beverages and the declining consumption of milk are of great public health significance for girls and women, because of their proneness to osteoporosis in later life."

Another study of high school girls published in a 2000 issue of "Pediatrics & Adolescent Medicine" showed a correlation between soft drink consumption and bone breaks. The study concluded that, "national concern and alarm about the health impact of carbonated beverage consumption on teenaged girls is supported by the finding of this study."

Because of the high content of phosphate in soft drinks, it lowers our calcium levels and raises the phosphate levels in the blood. When that happens the body in its infinite wisdom for survival pulls the calcium out of our bones. This is the reason that soft drink consumption can pose a significant risk factor for impaired calcification of growing bones principally in children.

According to the National Soft Drink Association (NSDA), consumption of soft drinks is now over six hundred 12-ounce servings per person, per year. Since 1978, soda consumption in the US has tripled for boys and doubled for girls. Young males, age 12-29 are the biggest consumers at over 150 gallons per year – that is about three quarts per week. At these levels, the calories from soft drinks contribute as much as 10 percent of the total daily caloric intake for a growing boy.

Beware of these ingredients in soft drinks:

High Fructose Corn Syrup - is associated with poor development of collagen in growing animals, especially in the context of copper deficiency. All fructose must be metabolized by the liver. Animals on high-fructose diets develop liver problems similar to those of alcoholics.

Aspartame - is used in diet sodas, and it is a potent neurotoxin (like rattlesnake venom) and endocrine (the system of the body that secretes hormones into the blood or lymph) disrupter.

Caffeine - stimulates the adrenal gland (which is situated above the kidneys and works to provide us with specific hormones) without providing nourishment.

Phosphoric Acid - added to give soft drinks "bite," is associated with calcium loss (and kidney stones, according to "Alternative Medicine," The Burton Goldberg Group).

Citric Acid - often contains traces of MSG.

Every time you pick up a soda, remember the following associated words:

Caffeine dependency
Obesity,
Weakened bones.

I had a patient complaining to me that he was having problems with his vision; this problem was affecting his overall daily activities. He had been to the eye doctor several times and they couldn't find anything wrong with his eyesight. I asked him what kind of medicine he was taking.

He gave me a list. One of his pain medications side effects produced blurred vision.

I told him if it was me I would try one week without taking the pain medecine and see what happens.

A week later he returned smiling, his vision had cleared, and to his amazement his pain was not any worse than when he was taking the "pain killers" as he called them.

You may ask what does taking prescription drugs have to do with soda pop, I am using this incident as an analogy of what happens to the body when you put in anything that affects health, be it soda pop, drugs, stress, the pollution in the air we breath, our thoughts, or food we partake that is unfit for human consumption.

Handy hints for household cleaning with Coca-Cola:

- Clean the toilet by pouring a can of Coca-Cola into the bowl. Let it sit for an hour, then flush it clean!

- To help get rid of some of the corrosion from car battery terminals, pour a can of Coca-Cola over the terminals.

- The corrosive ingredient in Coke is Phosphoric Acid which is a weak acid therefore it can't dissolve a nail, like you might have heard, but it can dissolve a tooth in about three days.

Most of our present health is in alignment to our way of life.

Sleep

If you want to see how much the spine benefits from a good night's sleep. Try this experiment: have someone measure your height upon getting up and then again before going to bed. You will notice that you are actually taller in the morning.

This restoration of the spine happens during the night, while you are sleeping, the time when the body takes a breather and puts to use some of its own healing power.

The National Sleep Foundation maintains that eight hours of sleep is optimal, claiming that it brings improved performance in tests, reduced risk of accidents and better immune system performance. Sleep is critical for proper function of the brain, immune system, endocrine system, (the secretion system), digestion, energy, recovery from injury, and restoration of health.

Contrary to the popular thought – "An hour of sleep before midnight is worth two after midnight," the most restful sleep you can get is early in the morning, according to Dr. Christian Guilleminault. If you can only get four or five hours of sleep, stay up as late as possible, to get the most benefit from your limited sleep.[1]

There are two types of insomnia. One has to do with difficulty falling asleep (sleep onset insomnia) and it is associated with anxiety or tension, pain or discomfort, and chemicals like caffeine and alcohol or simply fear of insomnia. The other type of insomnia is associated with frequent or early awakening (maintenance insomnia) and can be due to some serious health issues like depression, sleep apnea, drugs, alcohol, pain, or discomfort.[2]

Each year, four to six million people in the US receive prescriptions for sedative hypnotics (Narcotics). Psychological factors account for 50% of all insomnias evaluated in sleep laboratories.[2] But research published in the Archives of Internal Medicine as part of the large Wisconsin Sleep Cohort Study, states that sleep disorders are what's causing depression, and not the other way around.

This finding needs further research to be done since until now it has been common belief that difficulty with sleeping can be caused by some forms of depression.

• The word *apnea* comes from the Greek word meaning "without wind." Apnea is a temporary absence or pause of breathing. We all experience occasional pauses in breathing, that's perfectly normal, but when breathing stops for 20 seconds or more, it may easily disturb the sleep pattern by causing sleepiness after awakening in the morning, and tiredness and attention problems during the day. Obesity is the leading risk factor for sleep apnea and loud snoring [3,4]

The three most common symptoms of sleep apnea are: snoring, gasping for air and difficulty breathing while sleeping.

[1]Christian Guilleminault, MD, professor of psychiatry and behavioral sciences, Sleep Disorders Center, Stanford University, Stanford, CA

[2]Krammer, P. 'Insomnia: importance of the differential diagnosis', Psychosomatics, 1982, 23, pp.129-37.

[3]BidadK, Anari S, Aghamohamadi A, Gholami N, Zadhush S, Moaieri H. Prevalence and correlates of snoring in adolescents. Iran J Allergy Asthma Immunol. 2006 Sep; 5(3): 127-32.

[4]Lindberg E, Gislason T. Epidemiology of sleep-related obstructive breathing Sleep Med Rev.2000 Oct; 4 (5): 411-33.

Radiology class always started promptly at seven thirty in the morning. The teacher would pull the shades down on the only window in the classroom, and then turn off the lights. The idea was to make the room as dark as possible so that we got a more detailed picture of the X- rays being flashed on the screen. His voice was mellow, soft, seductive, and within a half hour of sitting at our desks staring at the dark "mysterious" slides, most of us would succumb to a state of natural rest.

An hour later the two gray metal doors opened to let in the blinding sunlight, like a lighthouse beacon shining into our dungeon. Feeling guilty but refreshed, I followed my fellow students into the next class across campus.

One day a miracle happened. One might even call it a revelation! A sleep expert came to one of our classes. After introducing himself as the "sleep doctor," he asked the class, "Are you having a problem staying awake during classes?"

None of us was going to admit to that. And then he quickly added, "Don't feel guilty about it! If you had slept enough the night before, you wouldn't be dozing off during the day. You are having problems staying awake during the day, because you have sleep deprivation!"

What a reality check! The idea that our tiredness during the day, and inability to concentrate in class or at work, could be taken care by going to sleep perhaps an hour or two earlier, suddenly became obvious.

We all know the answers to most of our problems, but sometimes we need to be reminded with outside reinforcement.

When I can't fall asleep because of something that happened during the day, and I find myself lying in bed rolling around from one side to the other, I get a flashback of my father saying, "The worst thing anybody can do is stay awake trying to solve a problem, because the next morning they will be too tired to do anything about it or even worse, they are too exhausted to remember what it was that kept them awake."

So I use some psychology by telling myself, "I really have a problem, that's true! But I better get to sleep or I am going to have to deal with falling asleep during the day over my paperwork, and not only that, but my face will look like it's been run over by an SUV." This train of thought has helped me more than a few times.

Some suggestions to improve sleep:

- Stay away from caffeine, (coffee, tea, cola and chocolate. Some prescription and non-prescription drugs contain caffeine) and nicotine (cigarettes and some drugs contain nicotine) at least 4-6 hours before going to bed. They are stimulants, therefore they can interfere with the ability to fall asleep.

- Try not to drink alcohol at least 4-6 hours before going to bed. Alcohol can make you drowsy, and help with sleep in the beginning because it slows brain activity but you will end up having fragmented sleep. Also, during the night after the body absorbs the alcohol, you will most likely wake up to go to the bathroom.

- Believe it or not, looking at the clock, if you happen to wake up during the night, can increase insomnia.

- Counting back from 100 may keep you awake, keeping track of the numbers. Try humming instead! Don't hum a tune - you may get so good at it that you won't want to stop ... Hum with a bored attitude, and feel yourself buzzing into sleep.

- Yogurt, bananas, figs, or turkey are naturally high on tryptophan, which acts as a natural sleep inducer. A turkey sandwich and a glass of milk as a snack before bed are sometimes recommended to help falling asleep.

- Make the bedroom your sleep sanctuary. No television, reading, or munching food in bed.

- Take a hot shower or a hot bath about an hour before bedtime. A hot bath will raise the body temperature, but the drop in body temperature is what may leave us feeling sleepy.

- No matter how bad the day goes, upon closing your eyes get in the habit of saying simple thanks, and acknowledging the close of the day.

- Choose a soft color for your bedroom walls. The green color is considered to convey an overall soothing, calm feeling and has even been attributed with healing powers. Green is often used in operating rooms by surgeons and staff. People waiting to appear on TV sit in "green rooms." Sage green is on the top of the list when it comes to giving humans a calm and natural feeling.

- Dressing the bedroom walls with pictures of places you would like to visit some day can give a dream-like feeling before closing the eyes.

- Decorate the bedroom with a few items from your past that tie with the present and bring you calmness and joy.

- Make sure the bedroom is dark and the windows have shades or curtains that are light proof.

- Keep the temperature in the bedroom no higher than 70 degrees. A hot room can be uncomfortable. Try a cooler room along with enough blankets to stay warm.

- Check out your medication's side effects. Is one of them keeping you "wired?" Talk to your doctor about it.

- If you have bad circulation and your feet get too cold during the night, it can keep you awake. Keep your feet warm by using soft, fleece socks.

- Check your mattress for sagging. Most people spend about one third of their entire life lying in bed. Make sure you have a good mattress. Get the best value and quality versus the price.

When I was in Salzburg, Austria in 1996, a friend asked me to treat her neighbor who suffered from constant back pain. I did an exam, and according to the findings I adjusted her back and neck. The next day she knocked at our door to tell me she felt great after the adjustment but that morning when she woke up she was once again in horrible pain.

My instincts made me ask, "Do you have a good mattress?"

And she said, "Yes, it's fine, not bad."

I politely asked her if she would mind I took a look at her bed.

"My mattress is about thirty years old," she said as she pointed to what looked more like a mine field after it had blown up. For anyone sleeping in that mattress, it was only a matter of time before they needed a chiropractor. Curiously enough her husband owned a mattress factory.

My son, Dr. Ralph, has told me several times that he misses the time when he was a "mobile" chiropractor. Going to a patient's home was very rewarding because it offered an open view of their living conditions and sometimes the culprit aggravating the symptoms.

Mattresses do not last forever. If good quality, they may last about 10 to 15 years.

Signs that a new mattress is needed:

- Waking up tired and achy because there isn't enough support being provided.
- Not comfortable during the night because the mattress sags, has lost its shape, or leaves an impression where you lie down.
- You tend to roll to the center or can't find a comfortable spot.
- Mattress looks worn or frayed.
- The box spring creaks and squeaks.

When you finally find a mattress you like, make sure they guarantee an exchange of mattresses if within a week or even a month you are not satisfied with the quality and how it's affecting your back or sleep.

* Night pain can also signify a serious health problem, which has nothing to do with your mattress. I always recommend a physical exam if the symptoms don't go away or are getting worse.

All mattresses are not created equal. Some tips on what to look for in a mattress:

Mattress type:

Don't let yourself be swayed by someone telling you what the best type of mattress is for them. As a chiropractor, I recommend you get a mattress that offers you the most support and is the most comfortable for you. If it is too firm, it won't support the body evenly, only the body's heaviest parts. If it is too soft and sags, then the spine can't maintain its natural curve. When sleeping, the spine will have less stress if it is supported and aligned the same as when standing. Try lying down on a few mattresses before settling.

A good nights sleep is essential for everyone. It is a time when our bodies and minds rest and rejuvenate. The spine works very hard all day supporting the body and its functions. Rest is essential to maintain this activity.

Box Spring:

It's a good idea not to mix a box spring (the foundation) with a different mattress. Getting the one that comes with the mattress you purchase can have a positive effect on the level of support and the durability of the mattress.

Pillows:

A water pillow is ideal for neck support, because you can use as much water as needed to fit your neck size while offering support to the neck contour and maintaining the natural curve as if standing, not allowing it to bend to one side more than the other.

**Dreaming
does not always make it so,
though with hope
we can keep it alive.**

Danlar

Smoking

"Once you start smoking, you will regret it for the rest of your life." This was an actual statement made by a 59-year-old patient who died from lung cancer, a year ago. Susan had been smoking since she was 16 years old. Some might think that dying at such an "old age" after smoking most of her life is not so bad. But she didn't just die. Her quality of life was depleted of the joy of living in the last few years, while going through chemotherapy in the hope of having another month added to her life.

This chapter on smoking is just a gathering of facts. Simply said, there are no eye openers or words of wisdom beyond what everybody has heard about or might know from personal experience. So, why bother? Because this book is about your spine and wellness, and as such it must address the most basic health issues that might influence the future of each reader.

- Tobacco use primarily begins in early adolescence. One third of all smokers had their first cigarette by the age of 14. Ninety percent of all smokers begin before age 21.[1]

- August 2006, a U.S. District Court judge found the tobacco companies guilty of civil racketeering charges for deceiving the public for more than 50 years. In her opinion, Judge Gladys Kessler also found that the companies continue to target kids, stating: "The evidence in this case clearly establishes that [companies] have not ceased engaging in unlawful activity…their continuing conduct misleads consumers in order to maximize [their] revenues by recruiting new smokers (the majority of whom are under the age of 18)…and thereby sustaining the industry."

There are two structures in the adult human body that lack blood supply, the cornea of the eyes which gets its nutrition from tears, and the intervertebral discs which depend on the nutrients from the end plate of the vertebral bodies. By smoking cigarettes, nicotine and carbon monoxide enter the body tissues by way of the blood stream and causes an adverse effect in the spine, by dehydrating the discs, which are supposed to be 85%, water. If you were already born with vertebral endplates or discs that are abnormal, smoking will cause the spine to degenerate faster. Smoking affects bones and joints, impairing the formation of new bone.

Would you buy a car without finding out the price and what the monthly payments are going to cost you?

When you start college, are you going to waste your time taking class after class without first consulting your counselor as to what subjects are most useful to give you entry into the profession you are looking for?

Before you take on a vice that will affect your future, shouldn't you talk to a few smokers and see what their life is like, living with addiction to tobacco?

[1]Mowery PD, Brick PD, Farrelly MC. Legacy First Look Report 3.Pathways to Established Smoking: Results from the 1999 National Youth Tobacco Survey, Washington DC: American Legacy Foundation, October 2000.

Tobacco smoking is associated with increased susceptibility to virtually every major chronic disease, here are a few with which most people are familiar by name:

Osteoporosis (Brittle bones)
Lung cancer
Stomach ulcers [2]
Periodontal disease and tooth loss - Tobacco smoking results in free radical damage, particularly to the surface cells of the gums. [3]
High blood pressure (Hypertension) [4]
Depression - smoking affects behavior through the actions of carbon monoxide (a known toxin to the brain) and nicotine and the induction of low vitamin C levels. [5]

A common visible symptom of smoking is premature aging of the skin, "the leather look." If maintaining a youthful appearance as long as possible is important, then appraising your present lifestyle is the key to prevention.

- The skin is the largest organ of the body in both surface area and weight. The skin is not just a thin coat that keeps the body together; it provides protection, regulates body temperature, detects sensation, and provides excretion and immunity by fending off foreign invaders. The skin's location makes it vulnerable to damage from trauma, sunlight, microbes and pollutants in the environment. Many interrelated factors affect both the appearance and health of the skin, including nutrition, hygiene, circulation, age, immunity, genetic traits, psychological state and drugs. Besides removing heat and some water from the body, sweat is also the vehicle for excretion of a small amount of salts and several organic compounds. [6] This fact alone, explains why when a long-term smoker leaves our office, we have to spray the treatment room with deodorizer to cover the offensive smell that lingers in the room after they have left.

Another side effect to smoking is the clogging of the arteries to the extremities [7] that can affect men later in life. It is clinically referred to as erectile dysfunction, which means the penis looses its normal sexual function by having difficulty with erection. No one can foretell how many years it takes to reach that stage, but when it happens, it will affect you physically as well as emotionally.

"It just stands to reason that what harms blood vessels in one area of the body harms them in other areas too," said Dr. David L. Katz, director of the Prevention Research Center at Yale University School of Medicine.

---

[2] Muller-Lissner, S. A., 'Bile reflux is increased in cigarette smokers,'Gastroenterol.,1986, 90, pp.1, 205-9.

[3] Christen, A., 'The Clinical effects of tobacco on oral tissue', J.A.D.A., 1970, 81,pp. 1,378-82.

[4] Kershbaum, A., Pappajohn, D., Bellet, S., et al., 'Effect of smoking and nicotine on adrenocortical secretion', J, A.M.A., 1968, 203, pp.113-16.

[5] Kinsman, R. and Hood, J., Some behavioral effects of ascorbic acid deficiency', Am.J. Clin.Nutr., 1971, 24, pp, 455-64.

[6] Gerard J. Tortora, Sandra Reynolds Graowski, 'Principles of Anatomy and Physiology" 7th Ed. The integumentary System. pp.127

[7] Smoking Causes Erectile Dysfunction through Vascular Disease. Shiri R. Hakkinen J. Koskimaki J. TammelaTL. Aurvinew University of Tampere, School of Public Health, Tampere, Finland (Urology 2006 Dec; 68(6):1318-22Epub Dec 4

Inhaling cigarette smoke means inhaling the following:

Nicotine - A colorless, poisonous alkaloid, derived from the tobacco plant and used as an insecticide.[1]

Carbon Monoxide - A colorless, odorless, highly poisonous gas, formed by the incomplete combustion of carbon.[1]

Tar - A dark, oily, viscous material consisting of hydrocarbons, produced by the destructive distillation of organic substances such as wood, coal, or peat.[1] Tar itself includes 4,000 chemicals. It is the main cause for lung and throat cancer, the effect is "smoker's cough," the yellow fingers and teeth, shortness of breath and wheezing.

Cyanide - Any of various compounds containing a CN group, especially the deadly poisonous compounds potassium cyanide and sodium cyanide.[1]

Benzene - A poisonous clear flammable liquid derived from petroleum and used in products such as insecticides and motor fuels.[1]

Formaldehyde - A poisonous cancer causing gaseous compound, used in aqueous solution as a preservative and disinfectant.[1] (Formaldehyde is useful in the preservation of cadavers, for dissection).

Methanol - A colorless, toxic, flammable liquid, used as an antifreeze, solvent, fuel, and denaturant for ethyl alcohol.[1]

Acetylene - A colorless, highly flammable or explosive gas, used for metal welding and cutting.[1]

Ammonia - A colorless, pungent gas, used to manufacture fertilizers and a wide variety of nitrogen-containing chemicals.[1]

"The risk of lung cancer is no different in people who smoke medium-tar, low-tar or very low-tar cigarettes," was concluded in a study led by Jeffrey E. Harris, professor in the economics department and in the Harvard-MIT Division of Health Sciences and Technology. This study was published in the British Medical Journal, 283 (1981)

- The Federal Government's National Cancer Institute (NCI) recently concluded that light cigarettes provide no benefit to smoker's health. Smokers crave nicotine, therefore they compensate by inhaling deeper, taking larger, more rapid or more frequent puffs, or smoke a few extra cigarettes to satisfy their craving. The end result is that smokers end up inhaling more tar, nicotine and other harmful chemicals.

- The NCI report concluded that strategies used by the tobacco industry to advertise and promote light cigarettes were intended to reassure smokers and to prevent them from quitting, and to lead consumers to perceive filtered and light cigarettes as safer alternatives to regular cigarettes.[2]

---

[1] The American Heritage Dictionary 4th edition. A Dell Book.pp. 573,134,838,217,82,335,534,7,28.
[2] National Cancer Institute. Risks Associated with Smoking Cigarettes with low Machine Measured Yelds of Tar and Nicotine. Smoking and tobacco Control Monograph 13.Bethesda, MD:NCI 2001.

Reanalysis of cigarette content confirms tobacco companies have increased addictive nicotine 11 percent over a recent seven- year period. The analysis was performed by a research team from the Tobacco Control Research Program at Harvard School of Public Health (HSPH) led by program director Gregory Connolly, professor of the practice of public health and Howard Koh, associate dean for public health for the Commonwealth of Massachusetts (1997-2003).

"Cigarettes are finely-tuned drug delivery devices, designed to perpetuate a tobacco pandemic," said former Commissioner Koh.

- Cigarette advertisements tend to emphasize youthful vigor, sexual attraction and independence themes, which appeal to teenagers and young adults struggling with these issues. A recent study found that 34 percent of teens begin smoking as a result of tobacco company promotional activities.[1]

- Another study found that 52 percent of smoker teens with non-smoking parents started smoking because of exposure to smoking in movies.[2]

Peers, siblings, and friends are powerful influences. The most common situation for first trying a cigarette is with a friend who already smokes.[3]

For every 100 sports physicals done to students between the ages 12 and 16 years old in our office, about 15% are smoking with their friends and or subjected to second hand smoke from their friends and or family members.

Second-hand smoke, is the combination of smoke emitted from the burning end of a cigarette, cigar, or pipe and smoke exhaled by the smoker.[4] Nicotine, carbon monoxide, and other evidence of second hand smoke exposure have been found in the body fluids of nonsmokers exposed to second hand smoke.

[1] Pierce JP, Choi WS, Gilpin EA et al. Tobacco Industry Promotion of Cigarettes and Adolescent Smoking. Journal of the American Medical Association 1998; 279(7): 511- 515.
[2] Dalton, MA.; Sargent, JD.; Beach, M.L.;et al. Effects of Viewing Smoking in Movies on Adolescent Smoking Initiation: A Cohort Study. Lancet 2003; 362:4999.
[3] U.S. Department of Health and Human Services. Preventing Tobacco Use Among Young People: A Report of the Surgeon General.1994.
[4] U.S. Department of Health and Human Services, Report on Carcinogens. 11th Edition. U.S. Department of Health and Human Services, Public Health Service, National Toxicology Program, 2005.

The tobacco companies are experts at reaching young people, because they know that they are most likely to become their lifelong customers. While visiting Turkey, I was shocked to see minors smoking cigarettes side by side with adults. The message was cleverly inscribed on some of their cigarette packages: "Be a real American, smoke American tobacco."

Even though most of the people in Europe and Middle East don't like American politics, they admire and envy our society in the sense that we are the powerful top dog, the boss and we are the only country in the world that offers the opportunity to be whatever one wants to be. They are enthralled by our music and our free style of living. They see it in the movies and on television, and they believe that to be our way of life.

Before I came to the United States, I was very much like them. I was convinced that I was going to see cowboys and indians still fighting in the prairies, and the rest of America consisted of Hollywood, New York, and movie stars. I believed that all Americans were millionaires, smoked, chewed gum and were impatient because they were more affluent than the rest of the world.

Smoking *American tobacco* in Turkey is the closest to being in America. Ironically, the Camel cigarettes in the US advertise, "Turkish tobacco is the world's smoothest, most aromatic leaf. Smoke the best. Smoke Turkish tobacco."

438.000 deaths – is the number of American deaths-per-year caused by smoking.

$13 billion – the amount Big Tobacco spends on promotions and advertising.

If these numbers don't add up, pretend you are a Big Tobacco executive; more than 400.000 Americans are dying from smoking every year – that's a lot of customers to replace. That's why, despite promises to stop, Big Tobacco continues to court new teen smokers to become its "replacement generation."

- American Lung Association

These are some of the strategies that might aid people who have already succumbed to the nicotine habit, and want to get help:

- Try not smoking today; tell yourself you can smoke the next day, if you make it through today. The next day, tell yourself the same. Take one day at a time. There are many addicts who successfully kicked their addiction of drugs like cocaine or heroin, by using this method. Of course you will feel irritable and stressed out, but that is perfectly normal. Kicking an addiction is never easy.

- Acupuncture has shown great success with addiction.

- Hypnosis can also be of helpful.

- For each day you don't smoke, put the money you would have spent, into a jar as a token of your daily commitment.

Sometimes it's easier to quit when you have help. If you want help, talk to your guidance counselor, school nurse, family doctor, or someone who has already quit smoking. Most people are not able to quit smoking the first time they try. The secret is not to give up. Do your best each time you try, eventually you will win!

For more information, and to get help for quitting smoking:

Nicotine Anonymous World Services.
Phone (866-536-4539)
http://www.nocotine-anonymous.org
The organization uses the same principles as Alcoholics Anonymous. It offers a directory of meeting places and times in many locations.

American Cancer Society.
Phone (1- 800-227-2345)
http://www.cancer.org and http://www.ca-journal.org
This organization offers a good program that covers four one-hour sessions during over a two-week period. They claim that 20% to 30% of people remain off cigarettes. Call to find out the nearest program for quitting smoking.

The American Lung Association.
(1-800-LUNG-USA) or (212-315-8700)
www.lungusa.org
This association is very responsive and offers a wide range of information and services.

SOURCES OF ALTERNATIVE METHODS:

American Academy of Medical Acupuncture.
(323-937-5514)
http://www.medicalacupuncture.org
To find an acupuncturist in your area (http://wwwmedicalacupuncture.org/refsearch.html)

The American Society of Clinical Hypnosis.
(630-980-4740)
http://www.asch.net
To find a reliable hypnotherapist send a self-addressed stamped envelope to the Society.

INTERESTING SITES:
This site provides tobacco company documents that have been produced from various lawsuits.
http://www.tobaccoarchive.com
http://www.smokefreekids.com/smoke.htm

Stress

Stress affects your spine, your muscles and your nervous system. Stress affects your overall health and without your health your life is less then adequate.

Our overall health can be affected by the on-going stress of modern life, such as peer pressure, keeping up with school, putting up with the boss, finances, long-term relationship problems, and other forms of constant stress.

Here is an example of ongoing stress, which can become chronic stress. There were two other students older than I at Life Chiropractic University, in Georgia. One of them was Mitchell; a man in his late 50's who literally dropped dead, while walking to one of his classes. Everybody that knew Mitchell stated that he was always too stressed and that was probably the reason he had died. After that happened, my friend Sara, who was 59 years old, told me she didn't care if the same happened to her, at least she was living her dream of being a chiropractor. And she was quick to add with a smile in her eyes, "If that happens, I won't have to pay my student loan!"

If I was not in school, I was at home studying into the wee hours of the night. I was an older student, English was my second language and I have a hearing deficit, which increased my problem, I knew I had to work harder than everyone else.

After studying all day Saturday, I got up early Sunday morning to continue my studies in preparation for a test early the next morning. It was about 11:00 when I felt a strange fluttering of my heart. I checked my pulse and so did my roommate who immediately offered to drive me to the emergency room. An exam was performed, and then they asked me to stay in bed and wait for the results. While waiting, I took the opportunity to go over my embryology book and the class notes, which I eagerly had taken along. When I looked up, the doctor was standing by the doorway staring at me. He pulled a chair and sat next to my bed.

"What are you doing?" He asked puzzled, as I had my notes all over the bed and was intensely looking over them.

"Studying for tomorrow's test," I answered, "I can't waste any time."

He gently took the book from my hand, and asked, "How long have you been in school?"

I answered, "Two years, and I have four more to go …"

He interrupted smiling and said, "I have good news, and bad news. First let me tell you the good news. There's nothing wrong with your heart. Now for the bad news, you are suffering from chronic stress and you are not going to make four years at the speed you are going." Then he gave me the best advice any doctor can give their patient, "If you don't take care of yourself and take one day a week to rest, you will soon return to this hospital, and I can't promise in what state of health you will be in. Take a walk in the park on Sunday. Go out for dinner or to a movie. Do something else besides consuming yourself with studying. Get a life! You will do a lot better when you take a test."

I thought about what happened to Mitchell, and decided to follow the doctor's advice.

"Stress is more prevalent than the common cold."

The American Medical Association

Five out of ten patients who come to our office for chiropractic care complain of stressful events prior to having back and neck ache, and or headaches. Stress affects the nervous system as well as the musculoskeletal system by interfering with the normal flow of energy throughout the body. Constant stress can cause health problems such as hair loss, depression, gum disease, high blood pressure, weight gain, weight loss, diabetes, muscular and joint pain, immune disorders, heart and digestive disorders. The list is almost endless when you consider that stress weakens the immune system.

Some causes of stress are temporary and part of daily living. A job interview, taking a driving test, waiting with someone for a baby to be born, looking for the first apartment ...These are what I call the fun stressors of living, the good stressors which can make life exciting.

Helpful suggestions for when you are having too much stress:

- Instead of taking a shower when you get home, try a hot bath with some Epsom salt added to the bath water.
- Take one day at a time.
- Do not extend yourself into more tasks than you can handle.
- Humor can help during difficult situations.
- Try reversing negative ideas by focusing on positive outcomes.
- Chiropractic care can help balance the spinal column and remove neurological interference (subluxations) caused by stress.
- Other ways to induce relaxation are acupuncture, massage, meditation, and deep breathing.
- *TESP* is a great way to let out frustrations.
- Sleep is important.
- Write a daily journal.

If you are taking meds, check out their side effects and consult with your physician before decreasing or eliminating them. Some antidepressants and other prescription drugs can harm you if stopped suddenly. Stress-inducing substances include some prescription drugs like analgesics, tranquilizers, antidepressants, sleeping pills, diet pills, muscle relaxants, anything with caffeine, tobacco, alcohol, marijuana and other so-called "recreational" drugs.

An inspiring approach for treating stress comes from Reinhold Niebuhr's notable prayer still used today at AAA meetings: "God, give us grace to accept with serenity the things that cannot be changed, the courage to change things that should be changed and the wisdom to distinguish one from the other."

If more than one thing in your life stresses you out, make a list and write down how you are going to manage them one by one. If it is impossible to do it on your own, talk to your parents, a counselor, a clergyman, or a friend whose advice you respect.

Depressed or aggressive mothers are often sources of stress in children, even more significant than poverty or overcrowding. Children are frequent victims of stress, because they are often unable to communicate their feelings accurately, or their responses to events over which they have no control.[1]

The first time I heard about psychotherapy was from Jessie, a student at Life University. We became good friends after attending a few classes together. One day she asked me if I would be willing to act as her psychotherapist, since her student budget no longer allowed such a luxury. She assured me that there was nothing to it; all I had to do was sit next to her and listen. But she did repeat several times, "I know it's going to be hard for you to keep quiet, but if the session is going to work, I need you to listen, and listen only!"

She would sit with a box of tissues on her lap and crying came easy for her, as she would tell me about her past and present frustrations. I knew she was doing better when she stopped crying and smiled, as she would always finish the "treatment" by saying, "Now let me share with you all the things I really should be thankful for."

After one year, I decided to transfer to another college, in California. The telephone became our long distance communication and she had no remorse calling me in the middle of the night, because she knew we were true friends.

"Hi, Veronica. Are you sleeping?"

Let's see, it's 2:00 in the morning. "Hi, Jessie, how are you? Yes, I am awake… you don't sound too good, what's going on?"

Her teary voice was always a dead give-away, "I need to talk to you. Do you mind?" And she would talk for about an hour, maybe more.

It was easy not to say anything, as I kept my eyes closed, listening.

From that experience I learned to encourage others to find a friend that will listen because as we hear our own thoughts out loud there is a better chance that we understand ourselves better. The healing comes from within ourselves; we just need a little push along the way.

---

[1] American Academy of Child and Adolescent Psychiatry, (202-966-7300)
www.aacap.org

National Institute of Mental Health. (301-443-4513)
www.nimh.nih.gov

American Institute for Cognitive Therapy (212-308-2440)
www.cognitivetherapynyc.com
Cognitive-behavioral Techniques include identifying sources of stress, restructuring priorities, changing one's response to stress, and finding methods for managing and reducing stress.

Simple instruction and information about a variety of meditation techniques.
www.meditationcenter.com

Osteoporosis

The reason I encourage every young person to read this chapter is because sooner or later we all get older, and the sooner we face the facts of our own mortality the better the chance we have to make the proper choices at a younger age. Getting older can be a wonderful experience if we stay active and healthy.

Osteoporosis is the result of gradual loss of both the mineral (inorganic) and non-mineral (primarily protein) portions of the bones. Osteoporosis literally means "porous bone." This weakening of the bones results in increased fractures, loss of height, back and hip pain and curvature of the spine.

We may be carrying our ancestors DNA and we may be prone towards diabetes, or arthritis, and so many other diseases that are beginning to run rampant in the USA, but I truly believe our health is a direct result of our life style. Two of the worst culprits are physical inactivity and poor diet. Start building your future now and create your own destiny, by making the proper choices.

Don't wait until your health starts to fail, or you look in the mirror and you don't like what you see. Start thinking like a Chiropractor and develop a philosophy based on prevention.

About 20 years ago when I was visiting my family in Lisbon, Portugal, my dad and I were in the grocery store when we ran into an old friend of his from Germany. She was a fragile old lady and she had an obvious curvature of the spine. He introduced me to her and she hugged me and held me for a while in her arms, as if she knew me and was glad to see me. She cried when she said, "If I had not been in a concentration camp, I could have had children, someone like you." She added, "The food they gave us was close to starvation. There was no nutrition for my bones or my female organs to grow. My period never came…but menopause did. The doctors have diagnosed me with osteoporosis, and told me I have curvature of the spine because I had no nutrition while growing up."

I felt sorry for her, but I didn't get the meaning of what she was telling me until I started writing this book. She was the ghost of the future, the future that awaits anyone that by choice or by force does not have the proper nutrition that the human body needs in order to be at its optimum.

It's not how long you live that is important, but how healthy you have lived that will produce the most impact throughout your life.

Wait one moment in your life.
Stop and listen to yourself.
Are your means
worth more than your health?

Danlar

In recent studies of younger people with Scoliosis, a strong connection has been found with osteoporosis or osteopenia.

Here are some interesting research findings I recommend you to read more about (check the internet, there are more available) since they link Scoliosis to loss of bone density:

- Research done at the Women's Medical and Diagnostic Center in Gainesville, Florida concluded that primary care physicians, especially gynecologists, can play a pivotal role by identifying women with higher risks for osteoporosis at earlier age; stressing the importance of developing maximal bone mass before menopause; and developing individualized patient prescription for bone mass determinants under personal control: exercise, nutrition (2.g., calcium and vitamin D), life – style, hormone replacement therapy.[1]

- According to the Department of Gynecology and Obstetrics, Cleveland OH. Amenorrhoea (a lack of menstruation) in female athletes is associated with both Scoliosis and fractures. Amenorrhoea is the result of low estrogen levels which is associated with osteoporosis.[2]

- In a study from the Department of Orthopedic Surgery, Louisiana State University Medical center, researchers concluded that of the females with Scoliosis in their study group, over one half were markedly osteoporotic.[3]

- Another study in the Journal of Pediatric Orthopedics found that adolescent girls with Scoliosis were found to have generalized state of osteoporosis.[4]

[1] Fertil.Steril. 1993 Apr; 59 (4): 707 – 25 "Osteoporosis: screening, prevention and management" Notelovitz M.

[2] Adolescent Med 1999 June; 10(2): 275-90,vii "Amenorrhea in the athlete" Gidwani GP

[3] J Pediatr Ortho 1992 Mar-Apr; 12 (2); 235-40 "Lumbar spine and femoral neck bone density in idiopathic Scoliosis: a follow up study" Thomas KA,CookSD,Skalley TC, Renshaw SV, Makuch RS, Gross M, Whitecloud TS 3rd, Bennett JT.

[4] J Pediatric Orthop. 1987 Mar-Apr; 7 (2):168-74 Trabecular bone mineral density in idiopathic Scoliosis. Cook SD, Harding AF, Morgan EL, Nicholson RJ, Thomas KA, Whitecloud TS, Rathen ES.

Known risk factors for females getting early onset of osteoporosis: (please note that where you find an *asterisk* the risk factor is extended also to males. Osteoporosis can affect both males and females)

    Early menopause
    Being female
* Advanced age
* Caucasian and Asian race
* Excessive use of alcohol
* Thin, small boned body type (Less than 127 pounds)
* Family history
* Smoking
* Medications (such as cortisone, Tagamet, some diuretics)
    Never been pregnant
* Inactive lifestyle
* Long-term use of anticonvulsants or corticosteroid therapy
* Hyperthyroidism
* Hyperparathyroidism
* A diet low in calcium and vitamin D
* High phosphorus intake (carbonated drinks)

Information and additional resources

National Osteoporosis Foundation
www.nof.org

The National Women's Health Information Center
www.4woman.gov

> **A mind clouded
> in negative thought,
> shades ambitions of good.
> Life
> *is* to entice happiness.**
>
> **Danlar**

Calcium

Contrary to what many people believe, osteoporosis is more than just a lack of calcium in the diet. It is a complex condition involving hormonal, lifestyle, nutritional and environmental factors.

Vitamins are not a substitute for food.

If you are allergic to dairy products, the primary source of calcium, you have other options.

Calcium from spinach is poorly absorbed, but kale is an excellent source of absorbable calcium and it is superior to milk. [1]

Precautions: Before using calcium supplements, consult your doctor if you have kidney stones, are taking diuretics, or have been diagnosed with high blood pressure.

Interactions with calcium: If you take calcium supplements don't take aspirin, erythromycin (antibiotic), or bisacodyl (for stomach ailments) because the combination of these meds with calcium can irritate the lining of your stomach and result in ulcerations.

The best form of calcium supplements: Calcium amino acid chelate or citrate. (Read the label of contents).

Least easily absorbed forms of calcium: Oyster shells and animal bones often in the form of calcium phosphate.

Calcium needs fats and oils in order to be absorbed therefore fat-free diets particularly in young women can result in early bone loss as well as ending ovulation. Both estrogen and progesterone can become decreased increasing a young woman's chance for early onset menopause.

The preferred type of fat needed in your diet for calcium absorption: fish and olive oil.

As we age the body doesn't produce as much hydrochloric acid in the stomach. **Not having enough acid in the stomach hinders the absorption of calcium.** Your naturopath physician can easily treat this condition.

99% of the calcium in our body is located in the bones and it is **the most abundant mineral in the body.**

Eskimos have a high incidence of osteoporosis due to their excessive protein-rich intake of meat and fish. Excessive intake of animal protein increases phosphate levels and changes the acid level in the blood causing calcium to be withdrawn from the bones, and then excreted in the urine.

Heavy consumption of phosphorous-rich foods cause calcium to be poorly absorbed, therefore check the labels of packaged goods and **avoid sodium phosphate, potassium phosphate, phosphoric acid, pyrophosphate, and polyphosphate.** Processed cheeses are high in phosphorous.

The Recommended Daily Allowance (RDA) **of calcium** for pre-menopausal and postmenopausal women is 1000 to 1200mg.

Calcium Content of Selected Foods, in Milligrams per 3 ½-oz. (100-g.) Serving

Kelp	1093	Yogurt	120	Black currant	60
Cheddar cheese	750	Wheat bran	119	Dates	59
Carob flour	352	Whole milk	118	Green snap beans	56
Dulse	296	Buckwheat, raw	114	Globe artichoke	51
Collard Leaves	250	Sesame seeds	110	Prunes, dried	51
Kale	249	Olives, ripe	106	Pumpkin seeds	51
Turnip greens	246	Broccoli	103	Beans, cooked dry	50
Almonds	234	English walnuts	99	Common cabbage	49
Yeast, brewer's	210	Cottage cheese	94	Soybean sprouts	48
Parsley	203	Soybeans, cooked	73	Wheat, hard winter	46
Dandelion greens	187	Pecans	73	Orange	41
Brazil nuts	186	Wheat germ	72	Celery	41
Watercress	151	Peanuts	69	Cashews	38
Goat's milk	129	Miso	68	Rye grain	38
Tofu	128	Romaine lettuce	68	Carrot	37
Figs, dried	126	Apricots, dried	67	Barley	34
Buttermilk	121	Rutabaga	66	Sweet Potato	32
Sunflower seeds	120	Raisins	62	Brown rice	32

Source U.S.D.A., Nutritive Value of American Foods in Common Units, Agriculture handbook No.456

Calcium deficiency can result in softening of the bones, bone deformities and growth retardation. Muscle spasms and leg cramps can also be the result of calcium deficiency.

• Osteoporosis affects 25% of women and 15% of men

• Osteoporosis affects about 20 million Americans annually.

The best defense against osteoporosis is to start building healthy bones while you are young.

What you can do:

1. Have a bone density test done, if your X-rays show the presence of osteopenia (bone density loss) depending on results, you may need a referral for medication to help increase and preserve your bone density.
2. See your chiropractor on a regular basis to help restore normal joint motion, related neurophysiological function and reduce discomfort.
3. If you smoke, quit.
4. *TESP* and weight bearing exercise becomes top priority. Weight bearing exercise of 25 minutes per day is recommended in order to be beneficial to your bones. Resistance training activities that involve pushing or lifting your own body weight like, walking, speed walking, biking, aerobic dancing, swimming, and cross-country skiing are best. While training, it's best to work out under the supervision of a certified professional.
5. Include dark green vegetables in your diet.
6. Eat a balanced diet.
7. Decrease sugary foods. (Sugar increases calcium loss in the urine.) [1]
8. Decrease coffee, sodas, alcohol (promotes calcium loss).
9. Maintain adequate but not excessive protein intake.
10. Vegetarians have a lower incidence of osteoporosis. [2,3,4]

The Nutritional Bone Builders (discuss these with your physician)

Calcium
Vitamin D
Magnesium
Vitamin B6
Folic Acid
Vitamin B12
Boron

---

[1] Heaney RP and Weaver CM, Calcium absorption from kale. Am J Clin Nutr 51, 656, 657, 1990
[2] Thom J, Morris J, Bishop A, and Blacklock, The influence of refined carbohydrate on urinary calcium excretion. Br J. Urol 50, 459-464,1978.
[3] Ellis F, Holesh S, and Ellis J, Incidence of osteoporosis in vegetarians and omnivores. Am J Clint Nutr 25, 55-58,1972.
[4] Marsh A, et al., Bone mineral mass in adult lactoovovegetarian and omnivorous adults. Am J Clin Nutr 37, 453-456, 1983.

Vitamin D

Vitamin D is produced in our bodies by the action of sunlight on our skin.

Vitamin D deficiency can cause Osteomalacia (softening of the bones) resulting in spinal curvature.

Vitamin D deficiency is most likely to be seen in people who are home bound and do not get sunlight. This is seen often in elderly people living in nursing homes. The consequences are lack of bone strength, density, and joint pain.

Natural food sources for Vitamin D: cod liver oil, salmon, mackerel, herring, butter, egg yolks, dark green leafy vegetables, milk fortified with Vitamin D.

Be aware of interactions: Vitamin D is no exception, since it is highly involved in calcium metabolism. Your general present health has to be taken into consideration. Drugs like cholestyramine, Dilantin, and Phenobarbital, just to name a few, will interfere with the absorption of vitamin D.

Once again, it is very important to refrain from taking over-the-counter medication, vitamins, or what we call "natural" remedies, until you have seen your doctor first. Some "innocent" vitamins can cause toxicity and Vitamin D is one of them. A characteristic of Vitamin D toxicity is an increased blood concentration of calcium, which can lead to kidney stones.

I believe in having a healthy diet and making sure sunlight is part of our daily walk outside, then we don't need to take extra vitamin D to supplement our diet.

Sunshine on my shoulders - makes me happy.
Sunshine on the water – looks so lovely,
Sunshine almost always – makes me high.

- John Denver

Magnesium

Magnesium is as important as calcium for the treatment and prevention of osteoporosis. Women with osteoporosis have lower bone magnesium content than women without osteoporosis. [1,2]

- About 60% of the magnesium in the body is in bone.

Refined foods, meat and dairy products do not contribute much to our needed daily magnesium requirements of 350 milligrams per day for adult males and 280 milligrams per day for adult females. Other negative factors that reduce absorption or increase secretion of magnesium, besides dietary deficiency, are high calcium intake, alcohol, antibiotics, diuretics, and oral contraceptives.

Magnesium Content of Selected Foods, in Milligrams per 3 ½-oz. (100-g.) Serving

Kelp	760	Soybeans, cooked	88	Potato with skin	34
Wheat bran	490	Brown rice	88	Crab	34
Wheat germ	336	Figs, dried	71	Banana	33
Almonds	270	Apricots, dried	62	Sweet potato	31
Cashews	267	Dates	58	Blackberry	30
Molasses, blackstrap	258	Collard leaves	57	Beets	25
Yeast, brewer's	231	Shrimp	51	Broccoli	24
Buckwheat	229	Corn, sweet	48	Cauliflower	24
Brazil nuts	225	Avocado	45	Carrot	23
Dulce	220	Cheddar cheese	45	Celery	22
Filberts	184	Parsley	41	Beef	21
Peanuts	175	Prunes, dried	40	Asparagus	20
Millet	162	Sunflower seeds	38	Chicken	19
Wheat grain	160	Common beans	37	Green pepper	18
Pecan	142	Barley	37	Winter squash	17
English walnuts	131	Dandelion greens	36	Cantaloupe	16
Rye	115	Garlic	36	Eggplant	16
Tofu	111	Raisins	35	Tomato	14
Coconut meat	90	Green peas.	35	Milk	23

[1] Gallai V, et al., Magnesium content of mononuclear blood cells in migraine patients. Headache 34, 160-165,1994.

[2] Cohen L and Kitzes R, Infrared spectroscopy and magnesium content of bone mineral in osteoporotic women. Isr J Med Sci 17, 1123-1125, 1981.

Pyridoxine (Vitamin B6)

A vitamin B6- deficient diet produced osteoporosis in rats; demonstrating that vitamin B6 plays an important role in bone health. [1] Besides its value in the treatment and prevention of osteoporosis, Vitamin B6 has been linked to boosting the immune system [2] and helping with asthma [3] depression [4] kidney stones [5] premenstrual syndrome [6] diabetes [7] and many other health conditions.

Be aware of Vitamin B6 interactions with food colorings, (especially FD&C yellow #5) and such drugs as penicillamine, Isoniazid, dopamine, hydralazine, oral contraceptives, alcohol, and excessive protein.

Most people don't believe it necessary to consult their physician when picking up a bottle of multivitamins, but it is very important to consult with your doctor because there's always a chance of your supplements interfering with the medications you are already taking. A naturopath physician should be considered.

Pyridoxine Content of selected Foods, in Milligrams per 3 ½-oz. (100-g.) Serving

Yeast, torula	3.00	Navy beans, dry	.56	Spinach	.28
Yeast, brewer's	2.50	Brown rice	.55	Turnip greens	.26
Sunflower seeds	1.25	Hazelnuts	.54	Peppers, sweet	.26
Wheat germ, toasted	1.15	Garbanzos, dry	.54	Potatoes	.25
Soybeans, dry	.81	Pinto beans, dry	.53	Prunes	.24
Walnuts	.73	Bananas	.51	Raisins	.24
Soybean flour	.63	Avocados	.42	Brussels sprouts	.23
Lentils, dry	.60	Whole-wheat flour	.34	Barley	.22
Lima beans, dry	.58	Chestnuts, fresh	.33	Sweet potatoes	.22
Buckwheat flour	.58	Kale	.30	Cauliflower	.21
Black eye peas, dry	.56				

[1] Benke PH, et al., Osteoporotic bone disease in the pyridoxine-deficient rat. Biochem Med **6,** 526-535, 1972.

[2] Beisel W, Edelman R, Nauss K, and Suskind R, Single-nutrient effects of immunologic functions. Jama **245,** 53-58, 1981.

[3] Collip PJ, Goldzier III S, Weiss N, et al., Pyridoxine treatment of childhood asthma. Ann Allergy **35,** 93-97, 1975.

[4] Russ C, Hendricks T, Chrisley B, Kalin N, and Driskell J, Vitamin B6 status of depressed and obsessive-compulsive patients. Nutr Rep Intl **27,** 867- 873,1983.

[5] Murthy M, et al., Effect of pyridoxine supplementation on recurrent stone formers. Int J Clin Pharm Ther Tox **20,** 434-437,1982.

[6] Berman MK, et al., Vitamin B6 in premenstrual syndrome. J.Am Diet Assoc **90,** 859-861, 1990.

[7] Jones CL and Gonzalez V, Pyridoxine deficiency: A new factor in Diabetic neuropathy. J Am Pod Assoc **68,** 646-653, 1978.

Folic Acid

Folic acid deficiency has been shown to cause changes in the blood chemistry of men and women by increasing homocysteine concentrations in the blood thereby interfering with collagen (the protein in the bone) cross-linking and leading to a defective bone matrix. The final result is osteoporosis.[1]

Folic Acid deficiency is linked not only with osteoporosis, atherosclerosis, and depression, but also with birth defects due to folic acid deficiency during pregnancy. The most common birth defect is spina bifida, which means the vertebrae failed to complete a protective ring around the spinal cord. The worst scenario is being born without the brain. Numerous studies have shown the benefit of folic acid supplementation beginning with preconception or very early on in the pregnancy and continued throughout [2, 3]

In a perfect world, it would be ideal for the mother-to-be to follow at least one year of good nutritional habits prior to getting pregnant. It is a known fact that folic acid is the most deficient vitamin in our diet due to people not eating enough "greens." A piece of lettuce on a burger or a side salad is not going to cut it. For a good source of folic acid, see below.

Folic Acid Content of Selected Foods, in Micrograms per 3 ½-oz. (100-g.) Serving

Yeast, brewer's	202	Lentils	105	Whole-wheat flour	38
Black-eyed peas	440	Walnuts	77	Oatmeal	33
Rice germ	430	Spinach	75	Cabbage	32
Soy flour	425	Kale	70	Dried figs	32
Wheat germ	305	Filbert nuts	65	Avocado	30
Liver, beef	295	Beets	60	Green beans	28
Soy beans	225	Peanuts	56	Corn	28
Wheat bran	195	Peanut butter	56	Coconut, fresh	28
Kidney beans	180	Broccoli	53	Pecans	27
Mung beans	145	Barley	50	Mushrooms	25
Lima beans	130	Split peas	50	Dates	25
Navy beans	125	Almonds	45	Blackberries	14
Garbanzos	125			Orange	5

[1] Gaby AR, Preventing and Reversing Osteoporosis. Prima Publishing, Rocklin, CA, 1994.

[2] Werler MM, Shapiro S, and Mitchell AA, Periconceptional folic acid exposure and risk of occurrent neural tube defects. JAMA **269**, 1257-1261, 1993.

[3] Milunsky A, et al., Multivitamin/folic acid supplementation in early pregnancy reduces the prevalence of neural tube defects. JAMA **262**, 2847-2852, 1989.

Cobalamin (Vitamin B12)

If you are a vegetarian you will need to supplement your diet with Vitamin B12, because Vitamin B12 is found only in animal foods (see below).

Folic Acid, vitamin B12 and Vitamin B6 are an important trio because of the interconnectedness of these three vitamins. It is therefore best to supplement with all three. [1,2]

Vitamin B12 Content of Selected Foods, in Micrograms per 3 ½-oz. (100-g.) Serving

Liver, lamb	104.0	Salmon, flesh	4.0	Blue cheese	1.4
Clams	98.0	Tuna, flesh	3.0	Haddock	1.3
Liver, beef	80.0	Lamb	2.1	Flounder, flesh	1.2
Kidneys, lamb	63.0	Eggs	2.0	Scallops	1.2
Liver, calf	60.0	Whey, dried	2.0	Cheddar cheese	1.0
Kidneys, beef	31.0	Beef, lean	1.8	Cottage cheese	1.0
Liver, chicken	25.0	Edam cheese	1.8	Mozzarella cheese	1.0
Oysters	18.0	Swiss cheese	1.8	Halibut	1.0
Sardines	17.0	Brie	1.6	Perch, filets	1.0

---

[1] Ubbink JB, et al., Vitamin B12, Vitamin B6, and folate nutritional status in men with hyperhomocysteinemia. Am J Clin Nutr **57,** 47-53, 1993.

[2] Ubbink JB, van der Merwe WJ, and Delport R, Hyperhomocysteinemia and the response to vitamin supplementation. Clin Invest **71,** 993-998, 1993.

Boron

The food source for Boron is fruits and vegetables. A diet rich in fruits and vegetables offers significant protection against osteoporosis and osteoarthritis.

Boron not only plays a major role in calcium and magnesium metabolism, but it is also necessary for the action of vitamin D, the vitamin that stimulates the absorption and utilization of calcium.

According to several large surveys, including the U.S. Second National Health and Nutrition Examination, fewer than 10 percent of Americans meet the minimum recommendation of two fruit servings and three vegetable servings per day, and only 51 percent eat one serving of vegetables per day.

Estrogen deficiency is associated with osteoporosis; however, estrogen supplementation has not been shown to actually increase bone mass, only slow down the progression of the disease. Before you decide to take estrogen look further into the side effects and the pros and cons to that decision, bringing up the fact that estrogen supplements has shown some conclusive side effects of cancer.

"There's no better investment a person can make than in one's health because the dividends pay off for a lifetime."

- Ralph Ezagui, DC

The Chiropractic Way

Be kind to your spine. Regular chiropractic adjustments will promote a healthy spine and nervous system.

Exercise for health. Perform *TESP* on a daily basis to improve your posture and strengthen your core muscles.

Choose not to smoke. For your personal health and for your loved ones. Tobacco has a negative effect on the bones, nervous system, lungs and heart.

Use a comfortable supportive mattress. For optimal spinal health sleep on your side or on your back, not face down, and plan for sufficient restful sleep.

Eat naturally. Avoid refined sweets, such as sodas and candy. Avoid saturated and trans fats usually found in fast food.

Drink water, at least 8 glasses of pure water every day.

Avoid drugs, including alcohol and caffeine.

Wear your book bag/backpack positioned on both shoulders for school, work or recreation.

Be a confident **"inner winner."** Hold your head high; keep your shoulders back.

Take time for relaxation and renewal. The stress of life impacts our health and posture.

Serve others. When you help someone and they want to pay you, ask them to pass it on instead. Kindness is a powerful gift that should be shared. It enhances the quality of our lives and our relationships.

Celebrate life as a learning experience. Learn from temporary setbacks and move on.

Practice thankfulness and positive thinking.

Read uplifting books.

Smile everyday, and the world around you will smile back.

The Quiet Corner

The purpose of the *Quiet Corner* is to help you find out more about yourself and allow you to make changes where you need, to make a difference in your life.

MY SURROUNDINGS

	True	False	Sometimes
I love where I live	_____	_____	_____
I know my neighbors	_____	_____	_____
I make my bed every day	_____	_____	_____
My bedroom is kept clean	_____	_____	_____
I keep my clothes clean and pressed	_____	_____	_____
My desk/work station is clean and inspiring	_____	_____	_____
I take part in helping to prepare the family meals	_____	_____	_____
I help my family/roommates to clean the house	_____	_____	_____
My homework is ready on time	_____	_____	_____
I am not a pack rat	_____	_____	_____
I recycle	_____	_____	_____

Concerning your surroundings, would you change anything, if you could?

Self Care

	True	False	Sometimes
I take a bath/shower every day	_____	_____	_____
I brush my teeth and floss every day	_____	_____	_____
I exercise daily at least 30 minutes	_____	_____	_____
I don't smoke	_____	_____	_____
I don't do drugs	_____	_____	_____
I don't drink	_____	_____	_____
I have my eyes tested every two years	_____	_____	_____
I visit my chiropractor regularly	_____	_____	_____
I visit my dentist every year for a check up	_____	_____	_____
I visit my Naturopath physician when I need nutritional counseling or an alternative to prescription drugs	_____	_____	_____
I visit my medical doctor once a year for my medical needs	_____	_____	_____
I do not indulge in overeating	_____	_____	_____
I don't eat when I am bored	_____	_____	_____
I don't reach into the refrigerator out of habit	_____	_____	_____
I sit and stand straight	_____	_____	_____

Do you have stress in your life? If so, what do you believe is the cause?

_____

_____

_____

_____

_____

_____

_____

_____

_____

_____

_____

_____

_____

_____

_____

_____

_____

_____

_____

_____

_____

_____

_____

_____

_____

_____

_____

_____

_____

_____

_____

_____

_____

_____

_____

_____

_____

_____

_____

_____

If your best friend was having the kind of stress you are experiencing, what advice would you give?

_____
_____
_____
_____
_____
_____
_____
_____
_____
_____
_____
_____
_____
_____
_____
_____
_____
_____
_____
_____
_____
_____
_____
_____
_____
_____
_____
_____
_____
_____
_____
_____
_____
_____
_____

From Inside Out

	True	False	Sometimes
I show respect to my parents /family/friends	_____	_____	_____
I do not gossip	_____	_____	_____
I accept who I am	_____	_____	_____
I stand by my word	_____	_____	_____
I am patient and a friend to my siblings	_____	_____	_____
I have a best friend	_____	_____	_____
I get along with everyone	_____	_____	_____
I do not judge or criticize others	_____	_____	_____
I use past experiences as learned lessons	_____	_____	_____
I lend a hand to the needy	_____	_____	_____
I have a life beyond school/work	_____	_____	_____
I never make self-doubtful remarks	_____	_____	_____
I am able to let go of unhealthy relationships	_____	_____	_____
I pass positive thoughts to others	_____	_____	_____
I don't dwell in the past or hold grudges	_____	_____	_____
I fall asleep looking forward to the next day	_____	_____	_____
I wake up smiling	_____	_____	_____
I am happy	_____	_____	_____

If there were no limits, what characteristics and traits do you see in the ideal you?

_____
_____
_____
_____
_____
_____
_____
_____
_____
_____
_____
_____
_____
_____
_____
_____
_____
_____
_____
_____
_____
_____
_____
_____
_____
_____
_____
_____
_____
_____
_____
_____
_____
_____
_____
_____

List the ten most important things in your life, starting with the most important five?

The Diary/Journal

I feel that a diary is more personal than a journal. A diary contains private thoughts and offers the freedom of expression without an audience. The inviting open pages are asking to be covered with words and eager to allow your inspiration to describe what you feel.

A journal is more like writing the day's event in a single blurt or a daily routine of thoughts, which is not really as private as a diary; you may not be comfortable with others reading what you have put down.

Try using the next pages to jot down your feelings and thoughts. It can be a short sentence, a long poem, or simply a story expressing how your day went. Record you future goals, your hopes and dreams, your greatest achievement. Learn from your past tragedies. This is your very private diary/journal. If you enjoy expressing yourself in the next two pages, get yourself a blank book to write in.

May your writing continue to grow like you are now, and let life inspire the poet from within.

And in Closing:

THE closing of a book.
Paper blues to best be described as
feelings and fears,
triumphs to depressing tears.
Words to be stabbed onto paper.
Last letters to be written,
or memory to share.
A new start but not an **END**

Danlar   (9-12-1987)

Credits

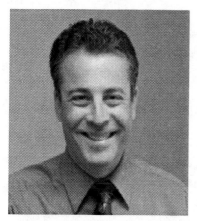

Dr. Ralph Ezagui – is a graduate of Western States Chiropractic College in Portland, Oregon. He was an adjunct professor at his alma mater for several years. He has his state licensure in Oregon, California and Washington. Dr. Ezagui has done radio interviews and written newspapers columns on the benefits of chiropractic care. When first practicing, he did house calls exclusively. Oregon's 12 was so taken by this that they aired a special segment on the nightly news in November of 1998 which included an interview. He has given numerous informational talks to the public and rarely turns down an opportunity to educate those interested in chiropractic. He is presently practicing in West Linn, OR. He has said, "To work side by side with my mother helping people recover or maintain their health is a powerful gift." www.gentledoctors.com

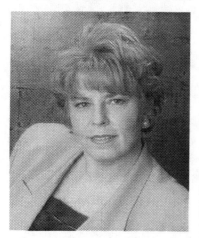

Dr. Pam Pavalonis – graduated from the National College of Naturopathic Medicine in Portland, Oregon in 2001, where she received her Doctor of Naturopathic Medicine degree. Dr. Pavalonis earned an MS degree, (majoring in hazardous materials) from ESF at Syracuse University and an MBA from Binghamton University in New York. Her favorite hobbies are cooking and gardening. She enjoys formulating the medicines she uses from the plants she grows. Her main office is in Portland, Oregon and she also works for a non-profit organization, Our House of Portland, a residential facility for people with HIV-AIDS.

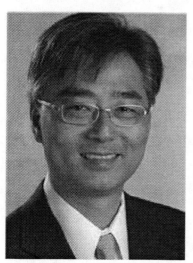

Dr. Tyrone Wei – received his Doctor of Chiropractic degree from Western States Chiropractic College (WSCC) and BS degree from the University of Oregon. He completed his residency in radiology at WSCC and is certified as Diplomate by the American Chiropractic Board of Radiology. Dr. Wei was formerly the Chairman of the Department of Radiology at WSCC. He held faculty positions at WSCC, National College of Naturopathic Medicine and Southwest College of Naturopathic Medicine. He is well published and lectured nationally. Dr. Wei maintains a full-time practice in radiology since 1983 in Portland, Oregon.

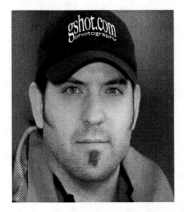

Dwon Güvenir – is an award winning photographer and photography instructor. He sits on the board of Directors of the Portland Metro Photographer's Association. He is a member of the National Association of Photoshop Professionals, Professional Photographers of America, and Nikon Professional Services. His images have appeared on TV, magazines, newspapers, busses, trains, and now books. He opened his studio in the Portland metro area in 2001 and has turned his passion for photography and teaching into a successful business. Visit www.oregonphotosafaris.com

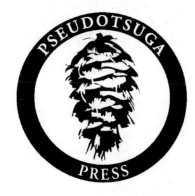

Chory Ferguson – provides copy and developmental editing services from his base in Portland, Oregon. He co-edits *Recto Verso* a literary magazine, and writes short fiction as a distraction from the rigors of real life. Often to be found slucking coffee from a stainless-steel mug at cafes in southwest Portland-red pen dutifully in hand—he enjoys the careful construction of dependent clauses, meticulous placement of em-dashes, and employment of passive voice. He may be reached by mailing chory@pseudotsugapress.com.

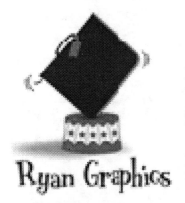

Ryan Graphics – was founded by Laurie Ryan-Day in 2001 shortly after finishing her graphic design degree. She is a freelance graphic designer that has shared her skills with freelance clients and various staffing agencies. Ryan Graphics is an award-winning graphic design firm that provides creative identity solutions for small-sized businesses. Other design services include identity package design, marketing collateral, packaging, illustration and production. For more information visit www.ryangraphics.com.

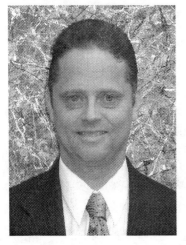

Danlar – is a professional artist in Portland, Oregon. His work has been called Abstract Organic because of the way he captures the Earth's innate beauty on canvas. He states, "My intent is to magnify the different depths and levels of matter into my paintings, photographs and sculpture."
Visit www.danlartartgallery.com

The Models

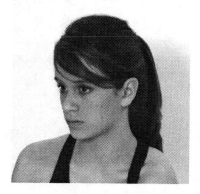

Molly – says she loves God and her friends. She enjoys all kinds of music, but her favorite is country. She has taken lessons in piano and voice for several years. Her favorite leisure activity is getting together with her friends.

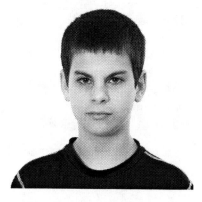

Connor – his favorite hobbies are sailing, fishing, skate boarding, rock climbing, listening to music, and eating home cooked meals. He enjoys especially, steak, fish and sushi. His favorite scouting activities are canoeing and sailing. He wants to attend college and become an environmental engineer.

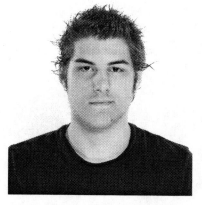

Josh – music, photography and filmmaking are his passions in life but he also enjoys skate boarding as a hobby. He plays all the instruments in his band, which he calls Cadet. His ambitions for the future are to make a living buskin, taking photos for bands, and making short films/music videos in Portland, Oregon and in N.Y. New York.

More about the Author

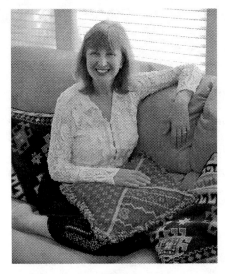

Dr. Veronica Esagui graduated from Life West Chiropractic College. She is licensed in Oregon, New Jersey and California. Born in Lisbon, Portugal, she speaks fluent Portuguese and Spanish. She came to the USA in 1962. Spending the first 30 years of her life in N.J., she raised two sons as she followed her passion for the arts by working as a guitar teacher, musician, newspaper reporter, television director, theatre producer and owner and manager of three music centers.

When she started Chiropractic College, her older son Ralph resigned from his position as an engineer at Bell Laboratories so that they might attend Chiropractic College together. She began the first year of school at Life Chiropractic University in Atlanta, Georgia, where she was awarded a full year scholarship for her work with the community. After one year, she transferred to Life College in California, where she graduated in December of 1997.

Over the years, Dr. Veronica Esagui is known for her own gentle adjusting technique, to help patients with Fibromyalgia. Upon trying to help Jean, one of her younger patients with Scoliosis, she created *TESP* a very specific protocol of exercises and stretches, which along with chiropractic adjustments proved to help.

Veronica's Diary – The Journey of Innocence the first of five books non-fiction sequel, will be released spring of 2009 followed by *Veronica's Diary II – Discovering the New World,* winter of 2009 in the US and internationally. To follow Dr. Veronica's book signings and events visit: www.veronicaesagui.com